Clinical Applications of Ayurvedic and Chinese Herbs

Monographs for the Western Herbal Practitioner

Clinical Applications of Ayurvedic and Chinese Herbs

Monographs for the Western Herbal Practitioner

by Kerry Bone

With technical and research assistance from Michelle Morgan

PHYTOTHERAPY PRESS

First Edition November 1996
Second printing May 1997
Third printing August 2000
Fourth printing April 2001

Published by Phytotherapy Press,
P.O. Box 276, Warwick, Queensland, 4370, Australia.

ISBN 0 646 29502 0

Typeset and designed by The Design Group,
Warwick, Queensland.

Printed by Printgraphics Pty Ltd, Blackburn, Victoria.

Preface

HERBAL MEDICINE is practised in every country of the world without exception. In fact, the World Health Organisation has estimated that more than 75% of the world's population still use the services of herbalists for the treatment of ill-health. Despite the plethora of different approaches, four great traditional systems of herbal medicine can be identified which incorporate the majority of people in the world. They are Ayurveda, Unani/Tibb, traditional Chinese medicine and its derivatives, and western herbal medicine.

Each of these great systems has a rich knowledge of life and philosophy, as well as disease states and plant medicines. There are some who feel that western herbal medicine is weak in philosophy, and it is true to some extent that the philosophical basis of western herbal medicine needs to be rediscovered. This rediscovery also represents an opportunity to develop western herbal medicine further, with inputs from science and the other systems. All major herbal systems are meeting the challenge presented by modern science. In fact, the governments of India and China are actively funding research on their medicinal plants. In the west, research funds come mainly from successful companies, especially those in Europe. All three systems are adapting to the times without losing sight of their traditional basis.

In early times, each herbal system was based around plants which grew in the immediate area. As trade increased, plants from more distant areas were incorporated. This fact is common to all the major systems. However, it is the western system which has incorporated more exotic herbs than any other system. With the trade in spices also came trade in medicinal plants. Plants which have been used for about a century or more in western herbal medicine include Rhubarb (Rheum) from Tibet, Ephedra and Panax from China, Jamaica Dogwood (Piscidia) from the Carribean, Chilli peppers (Capsicum) from South America and the Carribean, Kava (*Piper methysticum*) from the Pacific Islands, Echinacea and Hydrastis from North America, and Horse-chestnut (Aesculus) from northern India. These plants are household names to traditional western herbalists, yet their origins were originally regarded as exotic.

As the pharmacological and clinical information on exotic plants accumulates, largely funded by the governments of India and China, western phytotherapists face an important decision. Do they ignore this useful information, or do they attempt to incorporate these plants into their daily practice? However, there is no need for any soul-searching since a traditional precedent already exists. The western system has continually adopted herbs from exotic locations. As global communication reaches new heights, and the stresses of ever-increasing industrialisation create diseases common to all countries, modern phytotherapy must rise to the challenge. One aspect of meeting this challenge is the use of effective herbs, whatever their country of origin.

The purpose of this book is to provide comprehensive monographs on important Ayurvedic and Chinese herbs in a form which is suited to the practitioner of western herbal medicine. The monographs emphasize the large body of pharmacological and clinical information which is now available for these plants.

The monographs are intended as a useful tool for students and also for practitioners who wish to extend their therapeutic options.

Kerry Bone
October 1996

Contents

Chinese Herbs

Angelica sinensis

Mandarin	Dang Gui
English	Dong Quai
Family	Apiaceae
Part Used	Root

Properties

Sweet, acrid and warm. *Angelica sinensis* is a blood stimulant, menstruation corrective, laxative and builds blood. It is used for anaemia, menstrual problems, blood stasis and constipation. Different properties are ascribed to the head, tail and body of the root — the head is most tonic and the tail moves the blood most strongly. Such preparations are very expensive and the entire root is usually prescribed.

Active Constituents

Essential oil mainly consisting of ligustilide and n-butylidene phthalide.[1] The root also contains phytosterols, ferulic acid, fixed oil, and the coumarins angelol and angelicone. The high quality boxed root heads are extremely high in active constituents, e.g. ligustilide alone is 5.0%, which is more than 10 times the level in normal commercial roots.

Ligustilide

n-Butylidenephthalide

Pharmacology

→ *Effects on Sexual Function and the Uterus*

- The essential oil relaxes the isolated uterus, but other components increased uterine contraction.[1] Some experiments on the whole root have shown a stimulant effect *in vivo*, while others have shown that it can relax or co-ordinate (make more rhythmic) uterine contractions, depending on uterine tone.
- The root is devoid of oestrogenic action,[1,2] and its different parts have a similar effect on isolated rabbit uterus.
- One study showed increased sexual activity in female animals and a reduction in signs of vitamin E deficiency in male mice.[3]
- Butylidenephthalide demonstrated antispasmodic activity by inhibiting rat uterine contractions. Its action is non-specific similar to papaverine, but with a different mechanism of action.[4]

→ *Cardiovascular System*

- Dong Quai has a quinidine-like action on the heart. It can prolong the refractory period and correct experimental atrial fibrillation induced by atropine, pituitrin, strophanthin, acetylcholine or electrical stimulation.[1]
- Ferulic acid, is antiplatelet, as is the aqueous extract.[1]
- Dong Quai can prevent experimental coronary atherosclerosis in rabbits and rats.[1]

→ *Immunologic Function*

- Some studies have shown a pronounced inhibition of antibody production, while others have shown a sometimes weak stimulation of phagocytosis and lymphocyte proliferation.[1]
- Dong Quai can somewhat counter the immunosuppressive effects of hydrocortisone, but is not as effective as Astragalus.[5]
- Combined with Astragalus it improves thrombocytopaenic purpura in rabbits.

→ *Anti-inflammatory Activity*

- Tests on vascular permeability in mice showed an anti-inflammatory effect.[1] (This may partly explain its effects in dysmenorrhoea.)

→ *Other Effects*

- Feeding rats 5% Dong Quai for four weeks increased metabolism and oxygen utilization in the liver. Glutamic acid and cysteine oxidation were also enhanced.[3]

- Dong Quai increased red blood cell counts.[6]
- Ligustilide demonstrated a muscle relaxation effect in rats, believed to be of central origin.[7]
- Ligustilide demonstrated an antiproliferative effect on smooth muscle cells *in vitro*.[8]

Clinical Studies

- In combination with Corydalis, *Paeonia lactiflora* and Ligusticum, Dong Quai showed a 93% improvement rate for the treatment of dysmenorrhoea. The decoction was given daily, starting 5 days before and until cessation of menstruation. (After treatment for about 4 cycles, 72% were "cured".)[9]
- Ligustilide at 450 mg per day was used to treat 112 cases of dysmenorrhoea. The effective rate was 77% compared to 38% for aqueous extract of Dong Quai.[10]
- Infertility due to tubal occlusion was treated for up to 9 months with uterine irrigation of Dong Quai extract. 79% of patients regained tubal patency and 53% became pregnant.[11]
- Dong Quai has been successfully used to treat Buerger's disease and constrictive aortitis[1] and is often combined with Dan Shen in the treatment of angina, peripheral vascular disorders and stroke.
- Dong Quai reduced thymol turbidity in 88 cases of chronic hepatitis or liver cirrhosis (being a herb for blood stasis).[1]

Actions

Anti-inflammatory, regulates uterine function, antianaemic, antiplatelet, female tonic, mild laxative, antiarrhythmic.

Medicinal Uses

- Dysmenorrhoea, irregular menstruation, amenorrhoea, PMS, metrorrhagia, infertility, menopause. Often combined with Paeonia.
- Neuralgias and musculoskeletal injuries.
- Palpitations and cardiac arrhythmias, and cardiovascular disorders (with Dan Shen).
- Often combined with Astragalus for haematological immunological problems.
- Often used in combination for chronic liver disorders.

Contraindications

- Bleeding tendency or very heavy periods.

- First trimester of pregnancy.
- Tendency to spontaneous abortion.
- Acute viral infections such as colds or influenza.

Dosage

2 to 6g/day of the dried root, or 4 to 12 mL/day of 1:2 fluid extract.

REFERENCES

1   Chang H M and But, P P: *Pharmacology and Applications of Chinese Materia Medica*, Vol 2, World Scientific, Singapore (1987).

2   Lan, T H et al: *Acta Physiologica Sinica* **21**, 205 (1957).

3   Zhu, D P Q: *Am J Chin Med* **15**, 117 (1987).

4   Ko, W C: *Jap J Pharmacol* **30**, 85 (1980).

5   Luo, B et al: *J Beijing Medical Uni* **19**, 419 (1987) in *Abst Chin Med* **2**, 299 (1988).

6   Chang, H M: *Advances in Chinese Medicinal Materials Research*, World Scientific, Singapore (1985).

7   Ozaki, Y et al: *Yakugaku Zasshi* **109**, 402 (1989).

8   Kobayashi S et al: *Jap J Pharmacol* **60**, 397 (1992).

9   Liu, M A et al: *Beijing J Trad Chin Med* **5**, 30 (1988) in *Abst Chin Med* **3**, 61 (1989).

10   Gao, Y M et al: *J Lanzhou Medical College* **1**, 36 (1988) in *Abst Chin Med* **2**, 334 (1988).

11   Fu, Y F et al: *Jiangsu J Trad Chin Med* **9**, 15 (1988) in *Abst Chin Med* **2**, 422 (1988).

Artemisia annua

Mandarin	Qing Hao
English	Chinese Wormwood, Annual Wormwood
Family	Asteraceae
Part Used	Herb

Properties

Bitter and cold. Used for fevers, malaria, purpuric rashes and nosebleed.

Active Constituents

Artemisinin, a sesquiterpene lactone with a peroxide group which is a significant new antimalarial (also known as qinghaosu). The herb also contains an essential oil and flavonoids.[1,2]

Artemisinin

Pharmacology

➡ *Antimalarial Activity*

• Artemisinin and its derivatives are potent blood schizontocides.[1-3]

• The peroxide bridge in artemisinin and derivatives is essential for the antimalarial activity. Such compounds are thought to cause free-radical damage to parasite membrane systems.[4] Other natural peroxides have demonstrated anti-malarial activity, but in all cases were weaker than artemisinin.[5]

IN VITRO ACTIVITY

- Initial studies showed potent toxicity of artemisinin against chloroquine-resistant *Plasmodium falciparum*.[1]
- No marked cross resistance between chloroquine and artemisinin.[2]
- Flavonoids of Qing Hao potentiate the antimalarial effect of artemisinin,[6] particularly methoxylated flavones such as casticin and artemetin.[7]

IN VIVO ACTIVITY

- Oral administration of 50mg/kg artemisinin for 3 days cleared parasites from the blood of infected mice. Clinical studies in China and Vietnam verified this dose regimen to be optimum.[4]
- Since chemical derivatives of artemisinin are pharmacokinetically more available in the pure form, most studies now use these, and a broad spectrum of antimalarial activity has been demonstrated.[1,2,4]
- Artemisinin potentiates the toxicity of other antimalarials.[2,4]
- Resistance to artemisinin has been created in laboratory experiments, but develops at a slower rate than that for chloroquine.[2]
- In monkey malaria, a high relapse rate was observed which was reduced by combined treatment of Artemisia with Astragalus and Codonopsis.[2]
- Use of the whole herb demonstrates better potency than use of the pure chemical.[2]
- Gelatine capsules of *Artemisia annua* proved to be 3.5 times more effective than that of artemisinin for clearing parasitaemia in mice. The capsules were better than chloroquine in fever subsidence and removal of malarial symptoms. The recrudescent (re-infestation) rate was still high.[8]

NOTE:

- Despite the therapeutic benefits of artemisinin in treating malaria, widespread and uncontrolled use could result in side-effects, improper dose schedules and poor compliance. This, in turn, might cause treatment failure, recrudescence and possibly resistance to the drug.[9] Artemisinin is specific for the treatment of acute malaria, and may be unsuccessful for chronic malaria or as an antimalarial prophylactic.

➜ *Action Against Other Parasites and Organisms*

- Antischistosomal activity has been demonstrated in mice and rabbits for artemisinin.[2]

- A potent activity against *Clonorchis sinensis* was demonstrated in rats.[1]
- Artemisinin inhibited parasite growth in cultures of *Pneumocystis carinii*. High concentrations had no effect on feeder layer cells.[10]
- Artemisinin and derivatives demonstrated activity against *Leishmania major*, *in vitro* and *in vivo*. The compounds were effective by oral administration and injection.[11]
- The minimum inhibitory concentration of artemisinin was greater than 32 ug/mL against Gram-positive organisms (*Staphylococcus aureus*, *Streptococcus faecalis*) and the following Gram-negative organisms: *Klebsiella spp*, *Enterobacter spp*, *Shigella dysenteriae*, *E. coli*, *Serratia marcescens* and *Proteus spp*.[12]

➜ *Mechanism of Action*

- Artemisinin was observed to react with hemin and in the presence of red cell membranes this leads to the oxidation of protein thiols. As malarial parasites are rich in hemin, this may explain artemisinin's selective toxicity for the parasites.[13]
- The mechanism of action of artemisinin appears to involve two steps. In the first step, activation, intra-parasitic iron catalyses the cleavage of the endoperoxide bridge and the generation of free radicals. In the second step, alkylation, the artemisinin-derived free radical forms covalent bonds with parasite proteins.[14]

➜ *Immunologic Function*

- Artemisinin increases phagocytic activity but suppresses lymphocyte transformation.[1,15] Low doses may be immunostimulant but high doses are immunosuppressive and depress bone marrow function.
- Artemisinin and two synthetic derivatives demonstrated marked suppression of humoral responses in normal mice, but did not alter the delayed-type hypersensitivity response to mitogens. A selective immunosuppressive activity was demonstrated, which may be of benefit in the treatment of systemic lupus erythematosus (SLE).[16]
- Artemisinin and its water soluble derivatives demonstrated immunosuppressive action *in vitro* and *in vivo*.[17]
- Artemisinin and its derivatives enhanced T lymphocyte-mediated immune responses selectively in normal mice and accelerated immunoreconstitution of mice with bone marrow transplantation. These compounds may have application for the recovery of immune function.[18]

➡ *Cytotoxic Activity*

- Artemisinin demonstrated cytotoxic activity against several tumour cell lines *in vitro*.[19]

Pharmacokinetics

- A study revealed dihydroartemisinin to be the major early metabolite of several artemisinin derivatives. An artemisinin derivative, arteether was metabolized by two different isoenzymes of cytochrome P-450 in rat liver microsomes.[20]

- Animal studies using oral doses of artemisinin indicate it to have rapid absorption, wide distribution, rapid metabolism and excretion, and absence of accumulation.[2] Extensive first-pass metabolism is demonstrated. The half life of artemisinin is extended by its administration as a suppository.[4]

- In a cross-over trial by oral administration in humans, artemisinin was rapidly but incompletely absorbed. The mean residence time of intramuscularly injected suspension in oil was 3 times that of the oral formulation. The oral formulation requires more frequent administration. Injection and rectal administration of aqueous suspensions indicated a poor and erratic absorption.[21]

- Artemisinin has poor bioavailability and rapid elimination. In order to achieve adequate antimalarial plasma concentrations it is advisable to administer two oral doses of 500 mg per day.[22]

Toxicity

- Acute toxicity of artemisinin and its derivatives are low.[2] In animal tests, artemisinin compounds are considerably less toxic than quinoline antimalarials.[4] Artemisinin is not mutagenic but is teratogenic. However it has been used with pregnant women without adverse effects.[23]

Clinical Studies

➡ *Malaria*

- Since the early 1970's artemisinin has showed excellent activity against several forms of malaria, including those resistant to chloroquine. No serious side effects were observed. Early studies indicated a moderately high rate of recrudescent infection.[4] Radical cures came with higher doses.

- A suppository is a preferred method of administering artemisinin.[24]

- A randomized trial in Vietnam comprising 450 adults and children with acute falciparum malaria found a single dose of artemisinin in combination with an antimalarial drug (MSP) was effective in rapidly lowering parasitaemia and in preventing recrudescence. Adults received an oral dose and children received suppositories.[25]

- Early treatment of 21 cases of cerebral malaria with artemisinin (oral) resulted in 100% success in coma clearance after 14-21 hours, fever clearance after 54–97 hours and parasite clearance after 101 hours.[26]

- In an open clinical trial, artemisinin was observed to effectively influence the infectivity of gametocytes of *Plasmodium falciparum*. Artemisinin was much better at blocking the transmission of *P. falciparum* malaria than the antimalarial drug mefloquine.[27]

- A clinical trial conducted on over 1000 patients in Thailand observed artemisinin derivatives to be rapidly effective and safe. In combination with mefloquine the regime was highly effective against multi-drug-resistant *Plasmodium falciparum* infections.[28] Clinical trials in Vietnam have also observed effective treatment with drug-resistant *P. falciparum* malaria.[29]

- In a randomized clinical trial on 65 children with cerebral malaria, intramuscular administration of an artemisinin derivative produced shorter parasite clearance and coma times than did quinine.[30]

- In over 600 Vietnamese patients with *Plasmodium falciparum* or *P. vivax* malaria, recrudescence rates were highest (50%) in those receiving artemisinin for 5 days or less. For those receiving it for 5–10 days, a lower rate was observed (10–23%). Administration of tetracycline following artemisinin resulted in a 9.5% recrudescence rate.[31]

➜ *Lupus*

- Long term open studies in systemic lupus erythematosus (SLE) have seen a marked improvement after 50 days after use of 0.3g artemisinin per day (about 50 g of herb).[2]

- Another open study of discoid lupus used 36 to 54 g of herb per day, and remission was seen in 57% of patients.[2]

- One open study of discoid lupus used 6 pills of Qing Hao per day (dosage not specified) and skin lesions remitted in 6 of 8 patients.[32]

Actions

Bitter, antiparasitical, febrifuge.

Medicinal Uses

- Malaria and other parasitical infections.
- Systemic lupus erythematosus.

- Not advisable during pregnancy

 ## Dosage

10 to 20 g/day of the dried herb or 20 to 40 mL/day of the 1:2 fluid extract for an antiparasite effect. Higher doses may be needed in malaria, especially if not used in combination with longer lasting antimalarial drugs, or in severe cases. Higher doses may also be required for SLE. Lower dosages than this (eg. 3-10 mL/day) may be used for other conditions, such as improving immune function, jaundice, pruritus and low grade fevers.

REFERENCES

1 Tang, W and Eisenbrand, G: *Chinese Drugs of Plant Origin*, Springer Verlag, Berlin (1992).

2 Chang, H M and But, P P: *Pharmacology and Applications of Chinese Materia Medica* Vol 1, World Scientific, Singapore (1987).

3 Coleman, R E et al: *Acta Leidensia* **57**, 60 (1988).

4 Hien, T T and White, N J: *Lancet* **341**, 603 (1993).

5 Rucker, G et al: *Planta Medica* **57**, 295 (1991).

6 Li, K C-S et al: *Planta Medica* **55**, 654 (1989).

7 Elford, B C et al: *Trans Royal Soc Trop Med Hygiene* **81**, 434 (1987).

8 Wan, Y D et al: *J Parasitol Parasit Dis* (Engl) **10**, 290 (1992).

9 Arnold, K: *Trans Royal Soc Trop Med Hygiene* **88**, S47 (1994).

10 Merali, S and Meshnick, S R: *Antimicrob Agents Chemother* **35**, 1225 (1991).

11 Yang, D M and Liew, F Y: *Parasitol* **106**, 7 (1993).

12 Klayman D L et al: *J Nat Prod* **47**, 715 (1984).

13 Meshnick, S R et al: *Molec Biochem Parasitol* **49**, 181 (1991).

14 Meshnick, S R: *Trans Royal Soc Trop Med Hygiene* **88**, 31 (1994).

15 Wang, D R et al: *Shanghai J Immunol* **7**, 199 (1987) in *Abst Chin Med* **2**, 37 (1988).

16 Tawfik, A F et al: *Int J Immunopharmacol* **12**, 385 (1990).

17 Shen, M et al: *Scientia Sinica Series B* **27**, 398 (1984).

18 Yang S X et al: *Clin Immunol Immunopathol* **69**, 143 (1993).

19 Zheng, G Q et al: *Planta Medica* **60**, 54 (1994).

20 Leskovac, V and Theoharides, A D: *Comparative Biochem Physiol–C: Comparative Pharmacol Toxicol* **99**, 383 (1991).

21 Titulaer, H A et al: *J Pharm Pharmacol* **42**, 810 (1990).

22 Duc, D D et al: *Am J Trop Med Hygiene* **51**, 785 (1994).

23 Fu, L C et al: *J Trad Chin Med* **29**, 512 (1988) *in Abst Chin Med* **2**, 416 (1988).

24 Fan, T T et al: *J New Chin Med* **20**, 35 (1988) *in Abst Chin Med* **2**, 421 (1988).

25 Tran, T H et al: *Trans Royal Soc Trop Med Hygiene* **88**, 688 (1994).

26 Bui, D and Dinh, V B: *Bull Soc Pathologie Exotique* **86**, 500 (1993).

27 Chen P Q et al: *Chin Med J* **107**, 709 (1994).

28 Looareesuwan, S: *Trans Royal Soc Trop Med Hygiene* **88**, S9 (1994).

29 Hien, T T: *Trans Royal Soc Trop Med Hygiene* **88**, S7 (1994).

30 Taylor T E et al: *Lancet* **341**, 661 (1993).

31 Nguyen, D S et al: *Am J Trop Med Hygiene* **48**, 398 (1993).

32 Zhao, W F et al: *J Clin Dermotol* **16**, 126 (1987) *in Abst Chin Med* **2**, 187 (1988).

Astragalus membranaceus

Mandarin	Huang Qi
English	Milk-vetch Root
Family	Leguminosae
Part Used	Root

Properties

Sweet and slightly warm. Raises vitality, stops debilitating sweating, promotes healing and tissue regeneration. Good for organ prolapse.[1]

Active Constituents

Many constituents have been isolated from Astragalus root, but the relative importance of these constituents to oral activity in humans has not yet been clearly defined.

Many triterpenoid saponins have been identified including Astragalosides I to VIII, acetylastragalosides, astragenol etc.[2] The root also contains flavonoids, especially isoflavonoids which confer a yellow colour. A yellow colouration is traditionally regarded as an indicator of quality.

Polysaccharides have received considerable attention, especially the polysaccharide fraction F3. Plant sterols, a volatile oil and amino acids including GABA and *l*-canavanine have also been isolated from the root.[3] *Astragalus membranaceus* contains only very low levels of selenium since it is not one of the selenium accumulating species of the genus.

	R^1	R^2	R^3
Astragaloside I	Ac	Ac	H
Astragaloside II	Ac	H	H
Astragaloside IV	H	H	H

Pharmacology

➔ Immunity — Isolated Compounds

POLYSACCHARIDES

The polysaccharides show considerable immune-enhancing activity *in vitro*, but whether this always has relevance to oral use of Astragalus is open to question. Therefore for meaningful interpretation of the Astragalus research, data about whether the study was conducted *in vitro* or *in vivo* (and in the latter case the mode of administration) are essential.

Astragalus polysaccharides:

- potentiate the immune-mediated antitumour activity of interleukin–2 *in vitro*.[4]
- improve the responses of lymphocytes from normal subjects and cancer patients *in vitro*.[5]
- enhance natural killer (NK) cell activity of normal subjects and SLE patients *in vitro*.[6]
- and potentiate activity of monocytes *in vitro*.[7]
- F3 potentiated the lymphokine-activated killer-cell-inducing activity of recombinant interleukin-2 in cancer and AIDS patients *in vitro*.[8]

Astragalus polysaccharides are also active *in vivo* when given by injection:

- by intraperitoneal administration they increase the weight and cell number of the mouse spleen and stimulate phagocytic activity of peritoneal macrophages.[2]
- mice were protected against endotoxin after intraperitoneal administration of polysaccharide.[9]
- F3 given by intravenous injection countered the immune-suppressing effects of cyclophosphamide.[10]

SAPONINS

- Potentiate NK activity and restore steroid-inhibited NK activity *in vitro.*[11]
- Increase phagocytosis, bactericidal activity and acid phosphatase activity of peritoneal macrophages after sc injection.[12]
- Reduced nicotinic acetylcholine receptor antibodies in blood cell cultures from myasthenia gravis patients.[13]
- Demonstrated hepatoprotective effects on chemically-induced liver injury *in vitro* and *in vivo.*[14]

➜ *Immunity — Whole Root Extracts*

PHAGOCYTIC AND MACROPHAGE ACTIVITY

- Oral doses of decoction in mice for one to two weeks increased phagocytic activity.[15]
- Recently, oral doses of the dried root to growing mice enhanced phagocytic activity and increased superoxide production and acid phosphatase activity of peritoneal macrophages.[16]
- Ip administration of Astragalus and *Ligusticum lucidum* exerted an antitumour effect on renal cell carcinoma in mice, by improving phagocytosis and lymphokine-activated killer cell activity.[17]
- Astragalus reversed macrophage suppression induced by urological tumours *in vitro.*[18]

HUMORAL IMMUNITY

- Oral doses of dried extract given to humans increased levels of antibodies such as IgE and IgM.[15]
- Two months of oral treatment in subjects susceptible to the common cold greatly increased levels of IgA and IgG in nasal secretions.[15]
- A herbal formula containing Astragalus given in oral doses to mice raised serum IgG levels and the conversion percentage of lymphocytes. Resistance to the immunosuppressive effect of cyclophosphamide was also observed.[19]

CELLULAR IMMUNITY

- Oral doses of the dried root to growing mice significantly increased the proliferation of splenocytes induced by the mitogen concanavalin A.[16]

ANTIVIRAL ACTIVITY

- The antiviral action is most likely due to increased immunity and possibly enhanced interferon production.[15]
- Oral doses or nose drops of the decoction protected mice from infections with parainfluenza virus type I.[15]
- *In vitro*, Astragalus augments interferon response and acts synergistically with administered interferon.[15]
- Astragalus protects against Coxsackie B virus infection of myocardial cells *in vitro* and *in vivo* after ip injection.[20,21]

ANTITUMOUR ACTIVITY

- Shi-Quan-Da-Bu-Tang, (SQT) a Chinese herbal formula containing Astragalus and nine other herbs was selected as the most effective, potent biological response modifier after extensive screening of Chinese medicines. SQT shows immunomodulatory effects, potentiates therapeutic activity in chemotherapy and radiotherapy, prolongs survival and ameliorates adverse toxicities of many anticancer drugs. It also showed low toxicity.[22]
- Aqueous extract of Astragalus inhibited aflatoxin B1-induced mutagenesis in rat liver *in vitro*.[23]

➡ *Adaptogenic and Tonic Effects*

- Astragalus enhances cell growth, metabolism and longevity in cultures.[15]
- It improves survival in mice exposed to toxins and swimming stress.[1]
- Aqueous extract of Astragalus had a memory-improving effect on mice.[24]
- Astragalus lowered the collagen content in the aorta and lung of old rats to a level similar to that found in young animals.[25]

➡ *Cardiovascular System*

- Astragalus has a cardiotonic effect on isolated hearts and cardiac cells.[26]
- A cardiotonic effect was also demonstrated in heart failure patients.[27]
- Astragalus saponins have a positive inotropic action on the isolated working heart of rats.[28]
- A hypotensive action has also been observed, which may be due to cAMP elevation. GABA may be the active compound, but others have been proposed.[15]

➜ *Renal Function*

• Astragalus significantly reduced mortality and renal tubular necrosis in chemically induced renal failure.[29]

• Oral doses improve renal function in rats with experimental nephritis.[15] Large doses are traditionally used in the treatment of chronic nephritis.[15]

• A dose of 0.2g/kg in humans increased urine output by 64% and sodium excretion by 14.5%.[15] Oral doses also show activity as a diuretic in animal studies.

➜ *Other Effects*

• Water extract of Astragalus inhibited oxygen consumption caused by lipid peroxidation in isolated rat heart mitochondria.[30]

• Investigation into the effect of Astragalus on the activity of dog small intestine indicated it could strengthen the movement and muscle tonus, especially in the jejunum.[31] This activity supports its traditional use in organ prolapse.

• Water extract of Astragalus showed stimulatory effect on human sperm motility *in vitro*.[32]

Clinical Studies

➜ *Cardiovascular Conditions*

• Patients with heart failure due to vital energy deficiency were treated with Astragalus. Cardiac output and stroke volume were significantly increased. *Salvia miltiorrhiza* produced no effect.[33]

• Intravenous administration of Astragalus decreased erythrocyte sodium content and increased the sodium pump activity in a double-blind trial on patients with coronary heart disease.[34]

• Cardiac output increased in 20 patients with angina pectoris after treatment with Astragalus. There was however no improvement of left ventricular diastolic function.[35]

• Injection of Astragalus made the duration of ventricular late potentials shorten significantly in a trial conducted on cardiac patients.[36]

➜ *Immunologic Function*

• In an open study on 1000 subjects, a prophylactic effect for the common cold was shown for oral doses or a nasal spray. There was a decreased incidence and shortened duration of infection.[15]

• Patients with low white blood cell counts responded to treatment with Astragalus injection and levels were maintained above 4000 per mL in most cases.

- Patients with small cell lung cancer were administered combined treatment of chemotherapy, radiotherapy, immunotherapy and a herbal medicine consisting of *Panax ginseng* leaf and Astragalus root. The combined treatment raised the survival rates considerably, with some patients gaining 3 to 17 years of survival.[37]
- Injection of Ginseng-Astragalus used with chemotherapy in patients with malignant tumour of the digestive tract reduced the toxic effects of the chemotherapy and increased patient body weight. The white blood cell count was not reduced markedly, in contrast to controls.[38]

➜ *Other Conditions*

- Cases of chronic persistent hepatitis showed an 86% response rate after Astragalus injection.[15]
- Astragalus injection aids healing of peptic ulcers, especially gastric.[15]
- In a controlled double-blind study on 507 subjects, a combination of Astragalus with *Polygonum multiflorum* and *Salvia miltiorrhiza* was found to have an anti-ageing effect after oral administration. There was improvement in vigour, strength, sleep, appetite, hair greying, vision, and cellular immunity. Serum lipofuscin was decreased. Total effective rate was 76.6% compared to 34.5% for placebo (p<0.001).[39]
- Baoyuan Dahuang decoction (a herbal formula containing Astragalus and four other herbs) was administered to patients with chronic renal failure. In comparison to orthodox drug treatment, patients taking the herbal formula experienced improvement in symptoms.[40]
- Man-Shen-Ling, a herbal formula containing Astragalus demonstrated therapeutic effects on chronic nephritis. Oral administration to patients resulted in a 91% effective rate in comparison to 67% in the control group. Improvement was observed in proteinuria, haematuria, renal function, oedema, anaemia and anorexia. No adverse effects on major organs was observed.[41]

Actions

Immunostimulant, tonic, cardiotonic, diuretic, hypotensive.

Medicinal Uses

- Prevention of infection, impaired immunity.
- Chronic bacterial or viral infections especially if combined with debility and spontaneous sweating, e.g. AIDS.
- Chronic Fatigue Syndrome.
- Chronic and autoimmune diseases, especially nephritis.

- Congestive heart failure.
- Peptic ulcers.
- High blood pressure.
- Not advisable in acute infections.

Dosage

2 to 6g/day of the dried root or 4 to 12 mL per day of the 1:2 fluid extract.

REFERENCES

1   Bensky D and Gamble A: *Chinese Herbal Medicine Materia Medica*, Eastland Press, Seattle, (1986).

2   Tang, W and Eisenbrand G: *Chinese Drugs of Plant Origin*, Springer-Verlag, Berlin (1992).

3   Katsura, E et al: *Hokkaidoritsu Eisei Kenkyushoho*, **33** 136 (1983).

4   Chu, D et al: *Chung Hsi I Chieh Ho Tsa Chih* **10**, 34 (1990).

5   Wang, D C : *Chung Hua Chung Liu Tsa Chih* **11**, 180 (1989).

6   Zhao, X Z et al: *Chung Kuo Chung Hsi I Chieh Ho Tsa Chih* **12**, 669 (1992).

7   Chu, D T et al: *Chung Hsi I Chieh Ho Tsa Chih*, **9**, 351 (1989).

8   Chu, D T et al: *Chung-Hua Chung Liu Tsa Chih* **16**, 167 (1994).

9   Wang, L X and Han, Z W: *Yao Hsueh Hsueh Pao* **27**, 5 (1992).

10 Chu, D T et al: *J Clin Lab Immunol* **25**, 125 (1988).

11 You, L et al: *Zhongguo Mianyixue Zazhi* **6**, 60 (1990).

12 Chen, Y et al: *Zhongguo Yaolixue Yu Dulixue Zazhi* **2**, 305 (1988).

13 Tu L H et al: *Chin Med J* **107**, 300 (1994).

14 Zhang Y D et al: *Yao Hsueh Hsueh Pao* **27**, 401 (1992).

15 Chang, H and But P: *Pharmacology and Applications of Chinese Materia Medica*; Vol 2, World Scientific, Singapore (1987).

16 Sugiura, H et al: *Nippon Eiseigaku Zasshi* **47**, 1021 (1993).

17 Lau, B H : *Cancer Biotherapy* **9**, 153 (1994).

18 Rittenhouse, J R et al: *J Urol* **146**, 486 (1991).

19 He, J et al: *Hua-Hsi I Ko Ta Hsueh Pao* **23**, 408 (1992).

20 Yuan, W L et al: *Chin Med J* (Engl) **103**, 177 (1990).

21 Yang, Y Z et al: *Chin Med J* (Engl) **103**, 14 (1990).

22 Zee-Cheng, R K: *Meth Find Exp Clin Pharmacol* **14**, 725 (1992).

23 Wong, B Y et al: *Mutation Research* **279**, 209 (1992).

24 Hong G X et al: *Chung-Kuo Chung Yao Tsa Chih* **19**, 687 (1994).

25 Xu, P et al: *Chung-Kuo Chung Yao Tsa Chih* **16**, 49 (1991).

26 Li, S Y et al: *Acta Medica Sinica* 3, 27 (1988) in *Abst Chin Med* **2**, 303 (1988).

27 Zhu, B Q et al: *Chin J Integ Trad West Med* **7**, 591 (1987) in *Abst Chin Med* **2**, 159 (1988).

28 Wang, Q : *Chung Kuo Chung Yao Tsa Chih* **17**, 557 (1992).

29 Wang, Y J et al: *Chin J Nephrol* **4**, 217 (1988) in *Abst Chin Med* **3**, 41 (1989).

30 Hong, C Y et al: *Am J Chin Med* **22**, 63 (1994).

31 Yang, D Z: *Chung-Kuo Chung Hsi I Chieh Ho Tsa Chih* **13**, 616 (1993).

32 Hong, C Y et al: *Am J Chin Med* **20**, 289 (1992).

33   Zhu, B Q et al: Shanghai *J Trad Chin Med* **1**, 47 (1987) in *Abst Chin Med* **2**, 60 (1988).

34   Jin, C and Dai, R H: *Chung Hsi I Chieh Ho Tsa Chih* **11**, 651 (1991).

35   Lei, Z Y et al: *Chung-Kuo Chung Hsi I Chieh Ho Tsa Chih* **14**, 199 (1994).

36   Shi, H M et al: *Chung Hsi I Chieh Ho Tsa Chih* **11**, 265 (1991).

37   Cha R J et al: *Chung-Hua Nei Ko Tsa Chih* **33**, 462 (1994).

38   Li, N Q: *Chung-Kuo Chung Hsi I Chieh Ho Tsa Chih* **12**, 588 (1992).

39   Du, X et al: *Chin J Integ Trad West Med* **6**, 271 (1986) in *Abst Chin Med* **1**, 427 (1987).

40   Sheng, Z L et al: *Chung-Kuo Chung Hsi I Chieh Ho Tsa Chih* **14**, 268 (1994).

41   Su, Z Z et al: *Chung-Kuo Chung Hsi I Chieh Ho Tsa Chih* **13**, 259, 269 (1993).

Bupleurum falcatum

Bupleurum chinense can also be used.

Mandarin	Chai Hu
English	Hare's Ear Root
Family	Apiaceae
Part Used	Root

Properties

Bitter and cool. Bupleurum is diaphoretic, regulates gastrointestinal function and restores liver function. It is used to treat common cold, alternating chills and fever, liver enlargement, prolapse of the uterus and rectum, and irregular menstruation. Bupleurum is a major herb for the liver.

Active Constituents

Triterpenoid saponins (up to 2.8%)[1] known as saikosaponins a, b_1, b_2, b_3, b_4, c, d, e, f and polysaccharides (bupleurans).[2]

	R
Saikosaponin a	β-OH
Saikosaponin d	α-OH

Pharmacology

→ *Anti-inflammatory Activity*

- Oral administration of the saponins inhibit dextran-induced oedema in the rat paw.[1]
- Oral doses also suppress granulation tissue formation induced by croton oil.[1]
- Saikosaponins a and d stimulate and enhance adrenocortical function and this may produce the anti-inflammatory effect.[1]
- Intramuscular injection of saikosaponin d prevents the development of chemical-induced nephrosis.[3]
- Saikosaponins inhibit prostaglandin E_2 production *in vitro*.[4]

→ *Hepatoprotective Activity*

- Pre-treatment with saikosaponins markedly inhibits the acute and chronic toxic effects of many liver toxins such as carbon tetrachloride.[5]

→ *Effects on the CNS*

- The saikosaponins, when injected, are as potent as codeine in their antitussive effect.[1]
- Bupleurum has shown antipyretic action in several animal tests.[1]

→ *Effects on Digestive System and Metabolism*

- Oral doses of Bupleurum transiently increase blood glucose.[1]
- Oral administration increased bile output and bile salt content.[1]
- Oral administration of crude saponins or polysaccharides demonstrated anti-ulcer activity in animals.[2,4]
- Administration of Bupleurum to hyperlipidemic animals reduced cholesterol levels.[1,6]

→ *Immunologic Function and Antitumour Activity*

- Saikosaponin a and d demonstrated antitumour effects on human hepatoma cells *in vitro*.[7]
- Intraperitoneal administration of saikosaponin a, saikosaponin d and the aglycone of saikosaponin d (saikogenin D) demonstrated a marked increase in the number of macrophages in the peritoneum of mice. The activity of the aglycone suggests that oral doses of Bupleurum would stimulate macrophage activity.[8]
- A herbal formula, Sho-Saiko-To containing Bupleurum, *Scutellaria baicalensis* and five other herbs inhibited proliferation of human cancer cells *in vitro*,[9] and inhibited replication of HIV in lymphocyte cultures of virus-positive subjects.[10]

➔ *Other Effects*

- Saikosaponin a inhibited human platelet aggregation induced by ADP and dose-dependently inhibited thromboxane formation from arachidonic acid *in vitro*.[11]

Pharmacokinetics

- The saikosaponins undergo enterohepatic circulation and largely undergo faecal excretion. Oral doses are only one tenth absorbed compared to injected doses.[1]
- Evidence suggests saikosaponins are partly metabolized and hence a mixture of saponin, the monoglycoside and sapogenin is absorbed into the bloodstream after oral doses.[12]

Clinical Studies

- A clinical trial in chronic active hepatitis using oral doses of saikosaponins at a low dose of 6 mg/day (equivalent to about 0.3 g of root/day) showed remarkable reductions of serum liver enzymes, and results were statistically significant at 3, 6 and 12 months.[13]
- Satisfactory results were obtained in acute hepatitis. Is often combined with *Salvia miltiorrhiza* for chronic hepatitis with good clinical results reported.[1]
- Many studies have shown antipyretic effects in fever for more than 90% of cases.[1]
- Bupleurum given to patients with poor fluid excretion produced a diuretic effect.[1]
- In clinical study on 14 children with chronic hepatitis B virus infection and with sustained liver disease, Sho-Saiko-To (SST) promoted clearance of HBeAg.[14] *In vitro* studies indicated SST is able to modulate both cellular and humoral immune responses specific for hepatitis B virus-associated antigens.[15]

Adverse Effects

Bupleurum has a slight sedative effect in some patients and may also increase bowel movements and flatulence.[1]

Actions

Anti-inflammatory, hepatoprotective, antitussive, diaphoretic.

Medicinal Uses

- Acute and chronic liver diseases, chemical liver damage, poor liver function.

- Chronic inflammatory disorders, especially autoimmune diseases involving the liver or kidneys.

- Acute infections, common cold with chills and fever, chronic cough.

- Irregular menstruation.

- Often combined with Astragalus for debility and prolapse.

Dosage

1.5 to 6 g/day of dried root, 3 to 12mL/day of 1:2 fluid extract.

REFERENCES

1   Chang, H M and But, P P: *Pharmacology and Applications of Chinese Materia Medica,* Vol 2, World Scientific, Singapore (1987).

2   Yamada, H et al: *Planta Medica* **57**, 555 (1991).

3   Abe, H et al: *Eur J Pharmacol* **120**, 171 (1986).

4   Ohuchi, K et al: *Planta Medica,* p208 (1985).

5   Tang, W and Eisenbrand, G: *Chinese Drugs of Plant Origin*, Springer Verlag, Berlin (1992).

6   Mahato, S B et al: *Phytochemistry* **27**, 3037 (1988).

7   Motoo, Y and Sawabu, N: *Cancer Lett* **86**, 91 (1994).

8   Kumazawa, Y et al: *Int J Immunopharmacol* **11**, 21 (1989).

9   Yano, H et al: *Cancer Res* **54**, 448 (1994).

10   Buimovici-Klein, E et al: *Antiviral Res* **14**, 279 (1990).

11   Chang, W C and Hsu, F L: *Prostaglandins Leukot Essent Fatty Acids* **44**, 51 (1991).

12   Fujiwara, K and Ogihara, Y: *Life Sci* **39**, 297 (1986).

13   Hikino, H and Kiso, Y: *Natural Products for Liver Diseases*, in *Economic and Medicinal Plant Research* Vol 2, eds Wagner H et al, Academic Press (1988).

14   Tajiri, N et al: *Am J Chin Med* **19**, 121 (1991).

15   Kakumu, S et al: *Int J Immunopharmacol* **13**, 141 (1991).

Corydalis ambigua

Also known as *Corydalis yanhusuo*.

Mandarin	Yan Hu Suo
Family	Papaveraceae
Part Used	Rhizome

Properties

Bitter, slightly acrid and warm.[1] It is blood stimulant and analgesic and is used for organ pain, pain of injury, blood stasis and dysmenorrhoea.

Active Constituents

Almost 20 alkaloids have been isolated, including *dl*-tetrahydropalmatine (THP) and many other Papaveraceae type alkaloids.[2] THP and corydalis L are the most potent.[3]

Tetrahydropalmatine (THP)

Pharmacology

➡ Analgesic Action

- Analgesic potency of the rhizome is 1 to 10% that of Opium (depending on information source).
- Significant effects have been shown for the main alkaloids — 40% that of morphine.[1]
- THP and related constituents share a naloxone-resistant analgesic action and have no affinity for opiate receptors. (Naloxone is an opiate antagonist). They were recently found to be dopamine receptor antagonists.[4]
- Tolerance develops but at only half the rate for morphine. Cross tolerance with morphine was demonstrated.[5]
- THP is not addictive.[5]
- Corydalis strengthened the analgesic function produced by electroacupuncture in mice. The concentration of cytosolic free Ca^{2+} in two brain regions of treated mice was decreased.[6]

➡ Sedative Action

- THP has the main sedative action. Its hypnotic effect is mild and it antagonises caffeine and amphetamine.[3]
- THP significantly decreased motor activity of rats in a dose-dependent manner. Rigidity occurred at high dosage. The hypomotility produced by THP may be due to the increase in turnover rate of dopamine in the cortex and brain stem and of serotonin in the cortex.[7]

➡ Cardiovascular System

- The alcoholic extract is able to improve blood flow to the myocardium and may be of value in preventing heart attacks.[3]
- The extract also has antiarrhythmic action.[3]
- THP acts peripherally to lower blood pressure.[8]
- A drug based on THP was found to be effective and safe in treating patients with atrial fibrillation (especially paroxysmal atrial fibrillation).[9]
- Several alkaloids isolated from Corydalis showed protective effects on experimental myocardial infarction. THP and tetrahydroprotoberberines helped diminish myocardial infarction size within 24 hours and inhibited the rise in key enzymes within 4 hours.[10]

→ *Other Effects*

- The methanolic extract of Corydalis inhibited aldose reductase on rat lens *in vitro*. The aqueous extract was ineffective. Of the seven alkaloids isolated from the alcohol extract, only dehydrocorydaline inhibited aldose reductase.[11]

- Tetrahydroberberine, an alkaloid extracted from Corydalis, strongly inhibited platelet aggregation both *in vitro* and *in vivo* (by intraperitoneal and intravenous administration).[12]

- The methanolic extract of Corydalis was found to be effective in acute and chronic phases of inflammation by oral administration in rats.[13] *In vitro* work using the individual alkaloids confirmed this work.

- Protopine isolated from Corydalis was found to relax rat thoracic aorta mainly by suppressing the Ca^{2+} influx through both voltage and receptor operated calcium channels.[14]

- Results of receptor binding assay indicate that (–) THP is a dopamine receptor antagonist while (+) THP is a selective dopamine depletor. Intravenous injection of (–) THP to rabbits produced a marked analgesic effect but (+) THP did not.[15] Since Corydalis contains both isomers, both these activities can be expected.[3]

Pharmacokinetics

- Absorption of alkaloids is rapid and complete. Actions are rapid in onset but short-lived. The alkaloids cross the blood-brain barrier.[3]

Toxicity

- Oral administration of 1 to 50 mg/kg of gindarin (based on THP) to rats from the 1st to the 20th day of pregnancy demonstrated marked embryotoxic action.[16]

Clinical Studies

- THP has given analgesic effects in neuralgia, dysmenorrhoea and headaches. It has also been used to treat insomnia and hypertension.[3]

- The alcoholic extract of the root was successful in the treatment of angina pectoris and acute myocardial infarction, where the mortality rate dropped to 14%.[3]

Actions

Bitter, sedative, hypnotic, analgesic, cardioprotective, antiarrhythmic.

Medicinal Uses

- Almost any type of pain, in appropriate combinations, but especially visceral pain.
- Insomnia.
- Cardiac arrhythmias.
- Myocardial ischaemia.
- Contraindicated during pregnancy.

Dosage

5 to 10 g/day of the dried rhizome for an analgesic effect (or 10 to 20 mL/day of a 1:2 extract).

2 to 6 g/day of the dried rhizome for other effects (or 4 to 12 mL/ day of a 1:2 extract).

REFERENCES

1   Bensky, D and Gamble, A: *Chinese Herbal Medicine Materia Medica*, Eastland Press, Seattle (1986).

2   Tang, W and Eisenbrand, G: *Chinese Drugs of Plant Origin*, Springer Verlag, Berlin (1992).

3   Chang H M and But P P: (eds): *Pharmacology and Applications of Chinese Materia Medica*, Vol 1, World Scientific, Singapore (1987).

4   Gou-Zang, J: *TiPS* **8**, 81 (1987).

5   Jin, G Z et al: *Acta Physiol Sinica* **30**, 67 (1978).

6   Hu, J et al: *Chen Tzu Yen Chiu Acupuncture Research* **19**, 55 (1994).

7   Hsieh, M T et al: *Chin J Physiol* **37**, 79 (1994).

8   Xing, S H et al: *Acta Pharmacol Sinica*, **15**, 92 (1994).

9   Wang, D J et al: *Chung-Kuo Chung Hsii Chien Ho Tsa Chih* **13**, 455, 451 (1993).

10   Xuan, B et al: *Acta Pharmacol Sinica* **13**, 167 (1992).

11   Kubo, M et al: *Biol Pharmaceut Bull* **17**, 458 (1994).

12   Xuan, B et al: Acta *Pharmacol Sinica* **15**, 133 (1994).

13   Kubo, M et al: *Biol Pharmaceut Bull* **17**, 262 (1994).

14   Ko, F N et al: *Japanese J Pharmacol* **58**, 1 (1992).

15   Zhu, X Z: *Memorias do Instituto Oswaldo Cruz* **86**, 173 (1991).

16   Arzamastsev E V et al: *Farmakologiia i Toksikologiia* **46**, 107 (1983).

Paeonia lactiflora

Mandarin	Bai Shao
English	Paeony, White Peony
Family	Ranunculaceae
Part Used	Root

Properties

Sour, bitter and slightly cold. It is said to nourish the blood and relieve spasms. Used for dysmenorrhoea, muscle cramping, dysentery, dizziness, blurred vision and spontaneous sweating.

Active Constituents

Paeoniflorin, benzoylpaeoniflorin, albiflorin, oxypaeoniflorin and pentagal-loylglucose together with paeonilactones A, B and C.[1] Paeoniflorin is a monoterpene glycoside having a unique cage-like skeleton and occurs at about 1–2% in the root.[1]

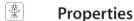

Paeoniflorin

Pharmacology — Paeoniflorin and Related Compounds

→ *Cognition Enhancement and Anticonvulsant Activity*

- Paeoniflorin, at an oral dose of 1 mg/kg in rats, attenuates the performance deficit produced by scopolamine in the radial maze.[2] The alpha 1-adrenergic systems are probably involved in this antagonising effect of paeoniflorin.[3] However, a later study suggested that peripheral beta 1-adrenergic systems are also involved.[4]

- Paeoniflorin at a very low oral dose (0.01 mg/kg) reduced learning impairment in aged rats.[5]

- Oral doses of albiflorin, pentagalloylglucose and aqueous extract of Paeonia inhibited the convulsant activity of the drug pentylenetetrazol in rats.[6]

→ *Influence on Steroid Hormone Function*

- Paeoniflorin bound minimally to oestrogen and androgen receptors, but not to progesterone receptor in human cytosol.[7]

- Paeoniflorin exhibited a moderate binding activity to glucocorticoid receptors in liver cytosol.[7]

- Paeoniflorin significantly decreased testosterone production from rat ovary *in vitro*. Results suggested that paeoniflorin inhibits testosterone synthesis. Estradiol synthesis was not affected.[8]

→ *Muscle-Relaxant Activity*

- Paeoniflorin exhibited a hypotensive effect in guinea pigs, possibly due to peripheral vasodilation. Vasodilation of coronary and peripheral vessels was established in a later study.[9]

- Paeoniflorin exhibited smooth muscle relaxant activity in both rat stomach and uterus.[9]

- The anticholinergic activity of Paeony root and its components was examined *in vivo* to substantiate the presence of analgesic, spasmolytic and antidiarrhoeal properties. Paeony extract was active *in vivo*. Fractionation revealed that paeoniflorin was one of the active constituents with anticholinergic activity *in vivo*, but it was inactive *in vitro*.[10]

- Paeoniflorin and related compounds inhibit twitch responses of skeletal muscle to direct and indirect stimulation. This effect was potentiated by glycyrrhizin from Licorice and was confirmed *in vivo*.[9]

→ *Other Effects*

- Paeoniflorin demonstrated anti-inflammatory activity for oedema induced by carrageenin and prevented stress ulcer in the rat.[1]

- Paeoniflorin and related compounds demonstrated antiallergic activity through inhibiting experimental contact hypersensitivity and passive cutaneous anaphylaxis.[1]

Pharmacology — Whole Root

- The root decoction has only a mild antispasmodic effect in mice, rabbits and guinea pigs,[9] and gastrointestinal administration of high doses (about 15 g/kg) increased uterine contractile activity in rabbits.[11]

- Paeony was found to inhibit 9 types of common pathogenic bacteria. It also enhanced phagocytic activity of macrophages in normal mice ($p<0.001$) and increased T-lymphocytes in cyclophosphamide-treated mice ($p<0.001$).[12]

- The Japanese formula Saiko-keishi-to (SK) contains Paeony as a major component. This formula has been extensively studied for antiepileptic activity, including clinical trials.[13] Paeonia shows clear inhibitory effects on the bursting activity of snail neurons induced by pentylenetetrazol.[14] This model is interpreted to demonstrate anticonvulsant activity.

- Paeony reduces testosterone production from ovaries but not from adrenal glands.[15]

- A combination of Paeony and Licorice taken orally relieved diarrhoea caused by the drug cisplatin in rats.[16]

- Paeony exhibited significant antiatherogenic activity in cholesterol-fed rabbits.[17]

- Paeony has hepatoprotective activity.[18]

- It inhibits platelet aggregation and increases fibrinolytic activity.[19] It has also been shown to prolong prothrombin time.[19]

Pharmacokinetics

- Paeoniflorin and related compounds undergo extensive metabolism by human intestinal flora *in vitro*. The first step in this metabolism is the removal of the sugar from the glycoside. A large number of bacterial species from human flora were capable of metabolizing paeoniflorin.[20] This study emphasizes the importance of *in vivo* studies using oral doses in assessing the pharmacology of Paeonia and paeoniflorin, since the active form in the bloodstream may be bacterial metabolites.

Clinical Studies

➜ *Reproductive System*

- Paeonia and Licorice were used to treat dysmenorrhoea in patients with vital energy and blood stasis.[21]

- Eight infertile, hyperandrogenic and oligomenorrhoeic women were investigated for the lowering of serum testosterone levels and the induction of regular ovulation by a formula comprising Paeony and Licorice.[22] After the treatment period, serum testosterone levels had normalised in 7 patients, and 6 patients were ovulating regularly. Two of these 6 patients subsequently fell pregnant.

- A recent study specifically examined the effect of a Paeony and Licorice combination in polycystic ovary syndrome (PCOS). Thirty-four Japanese women with PCOS were treated daily with 7.5 g of the combination for 24 weeks. Serum testosterone and free testosterone levels were significantly decreased after 4 weeks. However after 12 weeks, testosterone was only lower in the patients who became pregnant. After 24 weeks, the LH to FSH ratio was significantly lower in the treated group.[23]

- A traditional Chinese formula containing Paeony, *Paeonia suffruticosa*, *Poria cocos*, *Cinnamomum cassia* and *Prunus persica* might act as a weak anti-oestrogen. In an open study on 110 premenopausal patients with fibroids (uterine myomas), clinical symptoms were improved in 90% of cases and the fibroids shrunk in about 60% of cases.[24]

➜ *Other Conditions*

- Paeonia combined with Licorice and fossilised mammalian tooth was used to treat 43 cases of epilepsy for 2 to 3 months. 48.8% of cases did not have a relapse in 5 years.[25]

- Paeonia and Dan Shen were used to treat erythematous skin diseases with an 83% success rate.[26]

- Paeonia, Ginseng and *Stevia rebaudiana* were used to treat angina with a 93% success rate in symptoms and a 53% improvement in ECG. Microcirculation was also significantly improved.[27]

Actions

Antispasmodic, mild skeletal muscle relaxant, anticonvulsant, anti-inflammatory, cognition enhancer, antiallergic, immune enhancing.

Medicinal Uses

- Smooth muscle spasm, especially dysmenorrhoea, angina and migraine headaches.
- Muscle cramps, epilepsy.
- Polycystic ovary syndrome.
- Menstrual dysfunction, leukorrhoea.
- To assist memory.
- Often combined with Dong Quai or Licorice.

Dosage

2 to 6 g/day of the dried root or 4 to 12 mL/day of the 1:2 fluid extract.

REFERENCES

1   Tang, W and Eisenbrand, G: *Chinese Drugs of Plant Origin*, Springer Verlag, Berlin (1992).

2   Ohta, H et al: *Pharmacol Biochem Behav* **45**, 719 (1993).

3   Ohta, H et al: *Japan J Pharmacol* **62**, 199 (1993).

4   Ohta, H et al: *Japan J Pharmacol* **62**, 345 (1993).

5   Ohta, H et al: *Pharmacol Biochem Behav* **49**, 213 (1994).

6   Sugaya, A et al: *J Ethnopharmacol* **33**, 159 (1991).

7   Tamaya, T et al: *Acta Obst Gyn Scand* **65**, 839 (1986).

8   Takeuchi, T et al: *Am J Chin Med* **19**, 73 (1991).

9   Hikino, H: *Oriental Medicinal Plants* in Farnsworth, N R et al: (eds) *Economic and Medicinal Plant Research* Vol 1, Academic Press, London (1985).

10   Kobayashi, M et al: *Yakugaku Zasshi* **110**, 964 (1990).

11   Harada, M et al: *J Pharm Dyn* **7**, 304 (1984).

12   Liang, M et al: *New J Trad Chin Med* **21**, 51 (1989) in *Abst Chin Med* **3**, 274 (1989).

13   Abstracts of the *Satellite Meeting on Kampo Medicine* in conjunction with *10th International Congress of Pharmacology*, Auckland (1987).

14   Sugaya, A et al: *Planta Medica* **51**, 60 (1985).

15   Takeuchi, T: *Folia Endrocrinol Japon* **64**, 1124 (1988).

16   Xu, J D et al: *Chung-Kuo Chung Hsi I Chieh Ho Tsa Chih* **14**, 673 (1994).

17   Zhang, Y Z and Yan, X F: *Chung Hsi I Chieh Ho Tsa Chih* **10**, 669 (1990).

18   Qi, X G: *Chung Hsi I Chieh Ho Tsa Chih* **11**, 102 (1991).

19   Wang, Y and Ma, R: *Chung Hsi I Chieh Ho Tsa Chih* **10**, 101 (1990).

20   Hattori, M et al: *Chem Pharm Bull* (Tokyo) **33**, 3838 (1985).

21   Wu, Y X et al: *Shanghai J Trad Chin Med* p16, (1988) in *Abst Chin Med* **2**, 425 (1988).

22   Yaginuma, T et al: *Acta Obst Gynaec Japan* **34**, 939 (1982).

23   Takahashi, K and Kitao, M: *Int J Fertility Menopausal Studies* **39**, 69 (1994).

24   Sakamoto, S et al: *Am J Chin Med* **20**, 313 (1992).

25   Lin, W B: *Hunan Zhongyizazhi* p6, (1986) in *Abst Chin Med* **1**, 417 (1987).

26   Kong, Z et al: *J Trad Chin Med* **29**, 366 (1988) in *Abst Chin Med* **2**, 429 (1988).

27   Hu, J et al: *Chin J Integr Trad Western Med* **8**, 427 (1988) in *Abst Chin Med* **2**, 438 (1988).

Panax ginseng

Mandarin	Ren Shen
English	Chinese or Korean Ginseng
Family	Araliaceae
Part Used	Root; Red Ginseng is steamed before drying.

Properties

Sweet, slightly bitter and warm. Ginseng replenishes the vital energy, increases the production of body fluids and acts as a cardiotonic. Used for prostration, heart failure, asthma, dyspnoea, organ prolapse, diabetes, spontaneous sweating, cold limbs, palpitations, long-term debility and neurosis. Also used as a general tonic to promote health and longevity. It is said to benefit wisdom.

Active Constituents

The ginsenosides are considered to be the major pharmacologically active agents in Ginseng. These are dammarane saponins and can be divided into two classes — the protopanaxatriol class consisting mainly of Rg_1, Rg_2, Rf and Re and the protopanaxadiol class consisting mainly of Rc, Rd, Rb_1 and Rb_2. Ginseng root also contains other saponins, glycans and essential oils. Many other constituents have been identified.[1]

					% Content				
	Rg_1	Re	Rf	Rg_2	Rb_1	Rc	Rb_2	Rd	Total
Leaves	1.078	1.524	—	—	0.184	0.736	0.553	1.113	5.188
Leafstalks	0.327	0.141	—	—	—	0.190	—	0.107	0.765
Stem	0.292	0.070	—	—	—	—	0.397	—	0.759
Main root	0.379	0.153	0.092	0.023	0.342	0.190	0.131	0.038	1.348
Lateral roots	0.406	0.668	0.203	0.090	0.850	0.738	0.434	0.143	3.532
Root hairs	0.376	1.512	0.150	0.249	1.351	1.349	0.780	0.381	6.148

Table 1 Distribution of ginsenosides in *Panax ginseng*.

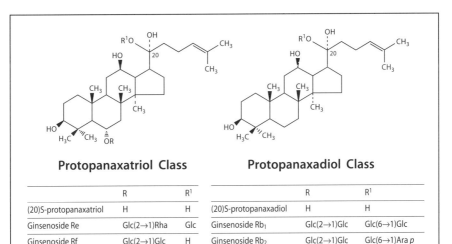

Protopanaxatriol Class **Protopanaxadiol Class**

	R	R¹		R	R¹
(20)S-protopanaxatriol	H	H	(20)S-protopanaxadiol	H	H
Ginsenoside Re	Glc(2→1)Rha	Glc	Ginsenoside Rb₁	Glc(2→1)Glc	Glc(6→1)Glc
Ginsenoside Rf	Glc(2→1)Glc	H	Ginsenoside Rb₂	Glc(2→1)Glc	Glc(6→1)Ara p
Ginsenoside Rg₁	Glc	Glc	Ginsenoside Rc	Glc(2→1)Glc	Glc(6→1)Ara f
Ginsenoside Rg₂	Glc(2→1)Rha	H	Ginsenoside Rd	Glc(2→1)Glc	Glc

Ara = α–L–arabinose, Glc = β–D–glucose, Rha = α–L–rhamnose, *f* = furanose, *p* = pyranose

Pharmacology

→ *Adaptogenic Action and Effect on the Pituitary-Adrenal Axis*

- Ginseng appears to act mainly on the hypothalamus and has a sparing action on the adrenal cortex, mediated through the anterior pituitary and ACTH release.[1]

- Ginseng increased cAMP levels in the adrenal cortex of rats.[2]

- Ginseng appears to tune the adrenal cortex so that phase 1 of the General Adaptation Syndrome (GAS) is more efficient. Response is stronger and quicker and feedback control is more effective so that when stress decreases, glucocorticoid levels fall more rapidly to normal.[3]

- During prolonged stress (or phase 2 of GAS) glucocorticoid production is reduced by Ginseng (a sparing effect), while at the same time adrenal capacity is increased (a trophic effect).[3]

- Ginseng also raises plasma ACTH and cortisone in the relaxed (non-stressed) state (thereby generating a sense of alertness and well-being).[4]

- In countless animal experiments, Ginseng has increases resistance to a wide variety of physical, chemical and biological stressors, e.g. it can reduce radiation damage.[1]

- The "diol" ginsenosides, particularly Rd, appear most active in activating the pituitary.[4]

- Ginseng can reduce blood glucose in hyperglycaemia, but increase it in hypoglycaemia.[5] Such normalising activity is characteristic of adaptogens.
- In normal fed rats, ginsenosides increased pyruvate kinase activity in the liver, but decreased it in high-carbohydrate-fed rats.[5]
- Ginseng has an antidiuretic action in mice, which is thought to be mediated via the posterior pituitary or increased mineralocorticoid synthesis.[1]
- Oral administration of ginseng root saponins or ginsenoside Rb_1 antagonized the immunosuppression induced by cold water swim stress in mice and rats. Conflicting results were obtained for serum corticosterone levels. The increase in serum corticosterone was inhibited in stressed rats, but accentuated in stressed mice.[6]
- Ginseng extract produced an increase in adrenal zona fasciculata cell size compared to controls. In animals treated with ginsenoside Rb_1 or Rg_1, the mean cell areas were unchanged but the distribution of cell sizes differed from controls.[7]

→ *Effects on Cellular Metabolism, Haematopoiesis and Blood Cells*

- Ginseng and ginsenosides stimulate DNA, RNA, lipid and protein synthesis in cells of liver, kidney, bone marrow and testes *in vitro*.[8]
- Ginseng promotes growth and longevity in tissue cultures of animal cells.[9]
- Ginseng increased red and white blood cells and haemoglobin in rabbits. Ginseng extract administered with food to mice was able to mitigate radiation damage to bone marrow.[10]

→ *Effects on Performance and Carbohydrate Metabolism*

- During exercise, Ginseng raises blood glucose and lowers circulating lactic acid and pyruvic acid. Plasma free fatty acids were also lowered.[11]
- Ginseng inhibits glycogen utilisation in skeletal muscle during exercise. Ginseng makes the muscle more able to use free fatty acids in the blood-stream, hence there is not as great a reliance on carbohydrate and glucose.[12]
- Ginseng improves oxygen uptake from haemoglobin in humans.[13]
- In human subjects, Ginseng improved muscle strength, recovery time and aerobic performance.[14]
- Students given 2 g of Jilin Ginseng per day showed improvement in red blood cell count, blood oxygen, haemoglobin, cardiac output and endurance.[15]

→ *Insulin Release and Blood Sugar*

- Ginseng exerts a mild hypoglycaemic action, but does not potentiate insulin.[5]
- Ginsenosides stimulate insulin release *in vitro*.[5]

- Recently, potent hypoglycaemic agents have been isolated including proteins and polysaccharides. Their oral activity has not been established.[5]

➜ *Hepatic Metabolism*

- Ginsenosides protect against carbon tetrachloride and galactosamine toxicity.[5]
- Ginseng accelerates ethanol metabolism in rats and humans and enhances blood alcohol clearance.[5]

➜ *Immunologic Function*

- Ginseng enhances phagocytosis and non-specific immunity, and increases natural killer cell and macrophage activity.[5]
- Ginseng enhances antibody formation *in vivo* but inhibits lymphocyte proliferation *in vitro*.[16]
- Oral doses of Ginseng enhanced B and T-lymphocyte activity in mice and increased interferon production.[17]

➜ *Mental Function and Performance*

- The total effect of the root is stimulatory, but the diols such as Rb1 are sedative and the triols such as Rg_1 are stimulatory.[18]
- Ginseng raised levels of amines in the brain except serotonin, which is decreased. Other studies have shown more complex effects. Blood-brain transport of *dl*-phenylalanine, a monoamine transmitter precursor, was promoted.[2]
- Oral doses of Ginseng (20 mg/kg for 3 days) improved learning and memory in rats and improved their sound and spatial discrimination.[19,20]
- The effect of oral doses of standardized extracts of Ginseng, Ginkgo and their combination were investigated on young and old rats in a series of behavioural tests. The effects varied with the dose and the test used, but both Ginseng and Ginkgo extracts demonstrated properties similar to nootropic drugs (drugs that affect neurons favourably). The two extracts and their combination improved the retention of learned behaviour.[21]
- After ongoing oral administration of Ginseng over five days, rats and mice showed positive results when tested in several anxiety models. These effects were comparable to those induced by injection of diazepam. Ginseng also attenuated the experimentally-induced decrease in rat brain MAO (monoamine oxidase) activity. This indicated an antianxiety effect.[22]
- Subchronic oral intake of aqueous extract of Ginseng inhibited the activity of nigro-striatal dopamine neurons in the daytime and activated spontaneous motor activity during the dark period in old rats, but produced the opposite effect in young rats. (Rats are nocturnal animals.)[23]

- Intraperitoneal administration of appropriate doses of Ginseng (ranging from 25 to 100 mg/kg/day) produced inhibition of the development of tolerance to morphine in rats.[24]
- Ginsenoside Rb_1 partially prevents the memory deficit induced by a cholinergic agent in rats. *In vitro* studies indicate ginsenoside Rb_1 has no effect on acetyl-cholinesterase activity, but facilitates the release of acetylcholine from hippocampal tissue. Its ability to prevent memory deficits may be related to facilitation of acetylcholine metabolism.[25]

➜ *Antitumour Activity*

- Ginseng inhibits the incidence and proliferation of tumours in mice exposed to carcinogens.[26]
- Ginseng promotes natural killer cell activity in mice with lung cancer.[27]
- Hepatoma cells cultured with ginsenosides appear to transform to normal cells (phenotypic reversion).[28]
- Ginsenoside Rh_2 exhibited significant induction of cell differentiation (pheno-typic reversion) of melanoma B16 *in vitro*.[29]

➜ *Sex Hormones and Sexual Function*

- Ginseng increases production of gonadotrophins *in vitro*.[30]
- Ginseng enhances the mating behaviour of male rats.[1]
- Ginseng induced a strong oestrogenic effect in oviarectomised rats.[1]
- It increases sperm count in rabbit testes and increases motility and prolongs survival of rabbit sperm.[1]
- In developing animals, Ginseng increases male and female sexual organ size. High oral doses of Ginseng in rats increase testosterone levels and reduce prostate size.[31]

➜ *Cardiovascular System*

- A study using isolated rat heart cells indicated Ginseng was able to delay experi-mentally-induced heart mitochondrial impairment and muscle contraction deterioration.[32]
- There appears to be no or slight cardiotonic effects in normal hearts, however a cardiotonic action was marked in heart failure.[1]
- Antiarrhythmic and myocardial protective effects have been shown, especially for ischaemia-reperfusion damage.[5]
- Intraperitoneal injection of ginsenosides decreased blood viscosity and platelet function in rabbits.[33]

Pharmacokinetics

- Oral absorption of ginsenosides is poor, but more are absorbed if administered as a mixture.[5]

- Administration of ginsenosides by injection to mice at first light dramatically raised serum corticosterone compared to administration at the beginning of darkness.[34]

- Ginsenoside Rg_1 is easily hydrated to its prosapogenin in the rat stomach. Ginsenosides Rb_1 and Rb_2 were hardly decomposed in rat stomach but were metabolized by enteric bacteria and enzymes. The amount of Rg_1, Rb_1, Rb_2 absorbed from the gastrointestinal tract was 1.9, 0.1 and 3.7% respectively. Rb_1 and Rb_2 were mainly excreted into the urine, Rg_1 mainly excreted via bile.[35]

- Further studies suggest the protopanaxatriol saponins undergo hydrolysis and hydration of the side chain while protopanaxadiol saponins undergo oxygenation of the side chain.[36]

Clinical Studies

➜ *Mental Performance*

- Ginseng improved competence, mood and performance of nurses on night duty.[37]

- Bulgarian research showed improvement in mental and nervous problems without adverse side effects.[38]

- In aged patients with problems of reduced intellectual output, loss of memory and slow thinking, the therapeutic effect of Ginseng was seen after one week with considerable improvement noted after two months.[38]

- In a double blind cross-over trial on university students, Ginseng improved performance of mental arithmetic.[39]

➜ *Cancer Therapy*

- 37 cases of chemotherapy-induced leukopaenia were treated with Ginseng. The treatment increased the white blood cell count to normal levels within two weeks in 82% of patients, without side effects.[40]

- Ginseng in combination with anticancer drugs shows definite therapeutic effects. Administration of Ginseng tablets for 30 days increased resistance to the adverse effects of antineoplastic medicines. The white blood count in patients increased by 65%.[41]

- An open clinical trial observed Ginseng to improve brain function and immune function in 127 cases of old age patients with cancer.[41]

- Prostisol, an extract of Ginseng root, demonstrated therapeutic effect on some tumours in clinical trials.[41]
- In a case-controlled retrospective study, Korean scientists found a significant reduction in overall cancer incidence with increasing Ginseng consumption. Ginseng extract or powder were shown to be more effective than the fresh root or the tea.[42]

➜ *Endrocrinologic Effects*

- Increases in sperm production in men and oestrogenic effects in middle-aged women have been noted.[43] In controlled trials, Ginseng has been shown to eliminate menopausal symptoms in a significant number of cases.[44]
- Ginseng and Licorice have been successful in treating Sheehan's syndrome and other causes of anterior pituitary hypofunction.[45]
- Blood glucose was lowered in mild diabetics.[1]

➜ *Cardiovascular Conditions*

- A clinical trial investigated the effect of Ginseng on thirty patients undergoing open heart surgery. Total ginsenoside or ginsenoside Rb was added to the cardioplegic solution. In comparison to controls, both ginsenoside solutions demonstrated protective effects on myocardial ischaemic and reperfusion injuries. Total ginsenoside produced a stronger effect than ginsenoside Rb.[46]

➜ *Other Effects*

- In Korea 120 patients with internal surgery were given Ginseng and showed improved liver function and weight gain.[43]
- One clinical study showed a reduction in blood cholesterol.[1]

Adverse Effects

Higher doses can overstimulate and aggravate insomnia, irritability, hypertension and cause tremor, euphoria, headaches, palpitation, decreased sexual function, morning diarrhoea, skin eruptions and menstrual abnormalities.

Actions

Adaptogenic, thymoleptic, stimulant, tonic, hypoglycaemic, immunostimulant, hepatoprotective, cardioprotective, antiarrhythmic.

Medicinal Uses

- Short-term use to cope with increased tiredness or stress or where increased mental or physical performance is required.

- To aid recovery from disease or surgery. To minimise the side effects of chemo-therapy or radiation.
- Angina, heart attacks and cardiac arrhythmias.
- To improve resistance to infection.
- Menopause.
- Impotence and poor sperm function.
- Anti-inflammatory due to its effect on endogenous glucocorticoids (combine with Licorice).
- Long-term use for the elderly and infirm as a tonic (lower doses).
- May be useful for diabetes, alcoholism, drug abuse, depression, mental disorders, asthma and cancer.

Contraindications

Acute asthma, hypertension, acute infections.

Dosage

0.5 to 3 g/day (depends on quality) of the dried main or lateral root or 1 to 6 mL of the 1:2 fluid extract. Preparations from the root hairs are therapeutically inferior and should be avoided. A ginsenoside ratio of Rg_1 to Rb_1 of greater than 50% indicates main and lateral roots have been used in product manufacture.

REFERENCES

1 Chang, H M and But, P P: *Pharmacology and Applications of Chinese Materia Medica*, Vol 1, World Scientific, Singapore (1986).
2 Fisel, J: *Arzneim-Forsch* **15**, 1417 (1965).
3 Fulder, S: *The Root of Being*, Hutchinson and Co, London, (1980).
4 Chang, H M et al (eds): *Advances in Chinese Medicinal Materials Research*, World Scientific, Singapore (1985).
5 Chen, X: *Abst Chin Med* **3**, 91 (1989).
6 Luo, Y M et al: *Chung-Kuo Yao Li Hsueh Pao* **14**, 401 (1993).
7 Buffi, O et al: *Bollettino-Soc Ital Biol Sperimentale* **69**, 791 (1993).
8 Yamamoto, M et al: *Arzneim-Forsch* **27**, 11 (1977).
9 Fulder, S: *Exp Geront* **12**, 125 (1977).
10 Yonezaka, M et al: *J Radiat Res* **26**, 436 (1985).
11 Avakian, E V et al: *Planta Medica* **50**, 151 (1984).
12 Avakian, E V Jr and Evonuk, E: *Planta Medica* **36**, 43 (1976).
13 Von Ardenne, M et al: *Panminerva Medica* **29**, 143 (1987).
14 McNaugton, L et al: *Int Clin Nut Rev* **9**, 32 (1989).
15 Jin, L S et al: *J Northwest Normal Univ* **2**, 137 (1986) in *Abst Chin Med* **1**, 410 (1987).
16 Jie, Y H et al: *Agents and Actions* **15**, 386 (1984).

17 Singh, V K et al: *Planta Medica* **50**, 462 (1984).

18 Shibata, S et al: *Chemistry and Pharmacology of Panax* in Farnsworth, N R et al: *Economic and Medicinal Plant Research* Vol 1 Academic Press, London (1985).

19 Petkov, V: *Arzneim-Forsch* **28**, 388 (1978).

20 Zhang, S C: *Chin Trad Patent Med* **11**, 29 (1989) in *Abst Chin Med* **3**, 151 (1989).

21 Petkov, V D et al: *Planta Medica* **59**, 106 (1993).

22 Bhattacharya, S K and Mitra, S K: *J Ethnopharmacol* **34**, 87 (1991).

23 Watanabe, H et al: *Jap J Pharmacol* **55**, 51 (1991).

24 Bhargava, H M and Ramarao, P: *Gen Pharmacol* **22**, 521 (1991).

25 Benishin, C G et al: *Pharmacol* **42**, 223 (1991).

26 Yun, T K et al: *Cancer Detect Prevent* **6**, 515 (1983).

27 Yun, Y S et al: *Cancer Detect Prevent Suppl* **1**, 301 (1987).

28 Odashima, S et al: *Europ J Cancer* **15**, 885 (1979).

29 Han, R: *Stem Cells* **12**, 53 (1994).

30 Li X M et al: *J Norman Bethune Univ Med Sci* **14**, 293 (1988) in *Abst Chin Med* **2**, 391 (1988).

31 Fahim, M S et al: *Arch Andrology* **8**, 261 (1982).

32 Toh, T T: *Am J Chin Med* **22**, 275 (1994).

33 Xu, Y J et al: *J Norman Bethune Univ Med Sci* **14**, 300 (1988) in *Abst Chin Med* **2**, 392 (1988).

34 Li, J C et al: *Acta Pharmacol Sin* **9**, 22 (1988) in *Abst Chin Med* **2**, 300 (1988).

35 Takino, Y: *Yakugaku Zasshi* **114**, 550 (1994).

36 Karikura, M et al: *Chem Pharm Bull* **39**, 400 (1991).

37 Hallstrom, C et al: *Comp Med East West* **6**, 277 (1982).

38 Popov, I M et al: *Am J Chin Med* **1**, 263 (1973).

39 D'Angelo, L et al: *J Ethnopharmacol* **16**, 15 (1986).

40 Zhou, J C et al: *Cancer Res Prev Treat* **14**, 149 (1987) in *Abst Chin Med* **2**, 323 (1988).

41 Liu, C X and Xiao, P G: *J Ethnopharmacol* **36**, 27 (1992).

42 Yun, T K and Choi, S Y: *Int J Epidemiol* **19**, 871 (1990).

43 Phillipson, J D: *Pharmaceut J* p161 (1984).

44 Yamamoto, M et al: *Am J Chin Med* **11**, 96 (1983).

45 Lei, C C and Tang, C C: *Chin Med J* (Engl) **11**, 156 (1973).

46 Zhan, Y et al: *Chung-Hua I Hsueh Tsa Chih* **74**, 626, 648 (1994).

Panax notoginseng

Also known as *Panax pseudoginseng*.

Mandarin	San Qi or Tian Qi
English	Tienchi Ginseng
Family	Araliaceae
Part Used	Root

Properties

Sweet, slightly bitter and warm. Tienchi stops bleeding, but transforms congealed blood, reduces swelling and alleviates pain and is indicated in haemoptysis, haematemesis, chest and abdominal pain, metrorrhagia, haematoma and in haemorrhage and pain caused by trauma.[1]

Active Constituents

Ginsenosides, many common to *Panax ginseng*, but with differing relative amounts. In China some of these saponins are called notoginsenosides but they may not be unique.[2]

Pharmacology

→ Cardiovascular System

- Tienchi increases coronary blood flow in many animal models.[3]
- It decreases myocardial oxygen consumption possibly through vasodilation.[3]
- Tienchi promotes collateral circulation to the ischaemic myocardium and protects against myocardial ischaemia and ischaemia-reperfusion damage in rats.[3]
- At high doses it appears to function as a calcium antagonist on myocardial function, but at lower doses may be cardiotonic.
- Panaxatriol exerted an antiarrhythmic effect in experimental models. A significant protective effect was observed towards atrial fibrillation.[4]
- Aqueous extract of Tienchi lowered systemic blood pressure in animals, an effect which was not blocked or reversed by multiple antagonists such as atro-

pine. It increased coronary blood flow after injection, without change in heart rate.[5]

→ **Effects on Blood Function**

- Tienchi shortened clotting time in rabbits and gave a good haemostatic effect in visceral bleeding.[3]

→ **Other Effects**

- Anti-inflammatory, anabolic, and androgenic effects have been observed.[6] Like Ginseng it increases protein synthesis.[2]
- The saponin fraction of Tienchi demonstrated anti-inflammatory, analgesic and immunomodulatory actions on experimental inflammation in mice after administration by injection. The effects of the saponins were similar to those of electroacupuncture which suggests that the saponin fraction might be an agonist of the opiod-like peptide receptor, but without addiction side effects.[7]
- Oral administration of the saponin fraction to animals for one week decreased their total cholesterol and triglycerides.[8]
- Ginsenoside Rg_1 isolated from Tienchi was effective in lowering hyperglycaemia and synergizing the action of insulin in normal animals. Synthesis of liver glycogen was increased. Its action in diabetic animals was dose-dependent, with no effect observed on insulin levels. The uptake of glucose by hepatocytes was increased *in vitro*.[9]
- Injection of a polysaccharide extract from the roots of Tienchi demonstrated strong reticuloendothelial system potentiating activity and enhancement of antibody production in challenged mice.[10]

Clinical Studies

- Many reports exist of satisfactory treatment in heart disease especially angina pectoris.[3]
- A haemostatic effect was achieved for haemoptysis in 5 days, and success has been noted in haematuria.[3]
- Eye drops were useful in haemostasis of the anterior chamber following surgery or trauma.[3]
- Tienchi was as effective as clofibrate in lowering cholesterol, but some scientists dispute this result.[3]

Actions

Antihaemorrhagic, cardioprotective, anti-inflammatory, antiarrhythmic, hypocholesterolaemic.

Medicinal Uses

- Internal bleeding, haemoptysis, haematuria, haematemesis, malaena and abnormal uterine bleeding.
- Myocardial ischaemia, arrhythmias, angina.
- High blood cholesterol.
- Traumatic injury especially with haematoma and bruising.
- May be useful for weight loss.
- Contraindicated in pregnancy.

Dosage

2 to 9 g/day of the dried root or 4 to 18 mL/day of 1:2 fluid extract. Higher doses for trauma and severe haemorrhage.

REFERENCES

1   Benksy, D and Gamble, A: *Chinese Herbal Medicine Materia Medica*, Eastland Press, Seattle (1986).

2   Tang, W and Eisenbrand, G: *Chinese Drugs of Plant Origin*, Springer Verlag, Berlin (1992).

3   Chang, H M and But, P P: *Pharmacology and Applications of Chinese Materia Medica*, Vol 2, World Scientific, Singapore (1987).

4   Gao, B Y et al: *Yao Hsueh Hsueh Pao* **27**, 641 (1992).

5   Lei, X L and Chiou, G C: *Am J Chin Med* **14**, 145 (1986).

6   Chen, Q S et al: *Bull Chin Materia Medica* **12**, 173 (1987).

7   Wang, Y L et al: *Chung-Kuo Chung Hsi i Chieh Ho Tsa Chih* **14**, 5, 35 (1994).

8   Xu, Q et al: *Chung-Kuo Chung Yao Tsa Chih* **18**, 367 (1993).

9   Gong Y H et al: *Yao Hsueh Hsueh Pao* **26**, 81 (1991).

10 Ohtani, K et al: *Planta Medica* **53**, 166 (1987).

Polygala tenuifolia

Mandarin	Yuan Zhi
English	Chinese Senega
Family	Polygalaceae
Part Used	Root

Properties

Bitter, acrid and warm. Polygala is beneficial to mental function, sedative and resolves phlegm.[1]

Active Constituents

Triterpenoid saponins including tenuifolin and a resin.[1,2] Polygala is chemically quite similar to the American Senega (*Polygala senega*).

Tenuifolin

Pharmacology

→ *Expectorant Action*

- Expectorant effect is a reflex caused by the irritant effect of the saponins on gastrointestinal mucous membranes.[1]

- The root bark is more expectorant than the root core.[1]

➜ *Sedative and Anticonvulsant Activity*

- Polygala has a synergistic action with barbiturates and antagonises chemically-induced convulsions.[1]

➜ *Antiageing and Neurological Activity*

- Oral doses of a Chinese prescription (DX-9386) containing Polygala, Panax, Acorus and Hoelen reduces impairment of learning and memory processes in learning-impaired mice. A sedative effect was also exhibited.[3]

- Chronic oral treatment of DX-9386 ameliorated the memory disorders in senescence accelerated mice. The herbal preparation reduced the elevated levels of lipid peroxide in the serum and liver of the animals. DX-9386 may have slowed the ageing process in terms of learning behaviour and lipid peroxidation.[4]

- An earlier study observed DX-9386 to prolong the life of senescence accelerated mice. The prescription prevented body weight decrease with ageing and tended to improved the senile syndrome.[5]

- DX-9386 enhanced long-term potentiation formation in the hippocampus of rats. The ameliorative effect of this prescription on learning-impaired animals may be due to its direct action on the hippocampus.[6]

- DX-9386 ameliorated the decreased learning and memory ability of thymectomized mice. Hypothalamic enzymes were normalised. The herbal treatment did not improve the reduced immune response.[7]

Clinical Studies

- Expectorant effects have been demonstrated.
- A herbal mixture containing Polygala has been successfully used for the treatment of chronic bronchitis and common cold with copious sputum.[1]

Actions

Expectorant, sedative.

Medicinal Uses

- Asthma, acute and chronic lower respiratory tract infections and catarrhal states.
- As a sedative, especially indicated for insomnia, palpitations, anxiety, restlessness. Is considered most effective in cases related to excessive brooding or constrained emotions.

Dosage

1.5 to 6 g/day of the dried root or 3 to 12 mL/day of the 1:2 fluid extract.

REFERENCES

1   Chang, H M and But, P P: *Pharmacology and Applicaitons of Chinese Materia Medica* Vol 1, World Scientific, Singapore (1987).

2   Tang, W and Eisenbrand, G: *Chinese Drugs of Plant Origin*, Springer Verlag, Berlin (1992).

3   Nishiyama, N et al: *Biol Pharmaceut Bull* **17**, 1472 (1994).

4   Nishiyama, N et al: *Biol Pharmaceut Bull* **17**, 1481 (1994).

5   Zhang, Y et al: *Biol Pharmaceut Bull* **17**, 866 (1994).

6   Zhang, Y et al: *Biol Pharmaceut Bull* **17**, 1337 (1994).

7   Zhang, Y et al: *Biol Pharmaceut Bull* **17**, 1199 (1994).

Polygonum multiflorum

Mandarin	He Shou Wu
English	Black-haired Mr He
Family	Polygonaceae
Part Used	Root which has been processed (Zhi He Shou Wu). Processing reduces toxicity and alters its properties.

Properties

Bitter, sweet, astringent and warm. Polygonum tones the vital essence and blood and fortifies muscles, tendons and bones. It is used in dizziness with tinnitus, premature greying, knee and low back pain and numbness of limbs.[1]

Active Constituents

Anthraquinones, tannins, phospholipids such as lecithin and is reputed to be rich in trace elements. Also contains tetrahydroxystilbene glucoside which may be the major active constituent.[1,2]

Pharmacology

➜ Blood Lipids and Atherosclerosis

- Prevents development of atherosclerotic lesions in rabbits fed cholesterol, but does not always lower cholesterol.[1]

➜ Antioxidant and Antiageing Activity

- Polygonum decreases levels of lipid peroxides in senile quails, and was more effective than Vitamin E in human tests. The life-span of senile quails was prolonged.[3,4]

- Polygonum antagonizes ageing through inhibition of a brain monoamine oxidase (MAO-B) and protects superoxide dismutase levels.[5]

- Polygonum inhibited oxygen consumption and malondialdehyde formation thereby demonstrating an inhibition of lipid peroxidation in isolated rat heart.[6]

→ *Other Effects*

- An extract of Polygonum demonstrated antimutagenic activity against benzo(α)pyrene *in vitro*. The extract also reduced the tumour incidence in mice.[7]
- Emodin isolated from Polygonum exhibited vasorelaxant and immunosuppressive effects *in vitro*.[8]
- Polygonum demonstrated an inhibitory effect on chemically-induced triglyceride accumulation in the liver of mice. Polygonum and its processed products reduced carbon tetrachloride-induced liver enlargement.[9]

Clinical Studies

- Dosages of 12g per day significantly lowered serum cholesterol in 62% of patients.[1]
- Good results were reported in nervous exhaustion with insomnia.[1]
- See also monograph on Astragalus.

Actions

Nervine tonic, antioxidant, antiageing, lowers cholesterol, bitter.

Medicinal Uses

- Neurasthenia especially with insomnia.
- Weak connective tissue.
- High blood cholesterol.
- Premature ageing.
- Tinnitus, dizziness and blurred vision.
- Promotion of longevity.
- Tonic for elderly.
- Possibly in nervous system diseases such as epilepsy, neuritis and schizophrenia.

Dosage

4 to 8 g/day of the dried root or 8 to 16 mL/day of 1:2 fluid extract. Higher doses for lowering cholesterol.

REFERENCES

1   Chang, H M and But, P P: *Pharmacology and Applications of Chinese Materia Medica* Vol 1, World Scientific, Singapore (1987).

2   Tang, W and Eisenbrand, G: *Chinese Drugs of Plant Origin*, Springer Verlag, Berlin (1992).

3   Wang, W et al: *Chin J Integ Trad West Med* **8**, 223 (1988) in *Abst Chin Med* **2**, 307 (1988).

4   Shi, T R et al: *Acta Med Sin* **4**, 104 (1989) in *Abst Chin Med* **3**, 154 (1988).

5   Deng, W L et al: *Chin Trad Herb Drugs* **18**, 138 (1987) in *Abst Chin Med* **2**, 84 (1988).

6   Hong, C Y et al: *Am J Chin Med* **22**, 63 (1994).

7   Horikawa, K et al: *Mutagenesis* **9**, 523 (1994).

8   Huang, H C et al: *Eur J Pharmacol* **198**, 211 (1991).

9   Liu, C et al: *Chung-Kuo Chung Yao Tsa Chih* **17**, 595, 639 (1992).

Rehmannia glutinosa

Mandarin	Di Huang
	If uncured is called Sheng Di Huang. If cooked with wine (cured) is called Shu Di Huang
English	Chinese Foxglove
Family	Scrophulariaceae
Part Used	Root

Properties

- Uncured Rehmannia is sweet, slightly bitter, cold. It is thought to be antipyretic, haemostatic and removes latent heat from the blood. It is used in skin rashes, diabetes, low grade fevers and bleeding.

- Cured Rehmannia is sweet and slightly warm. It regulates menstruation and promotes blood production and is used for anaemia, dizziness, weakness, tinnitus etc. (similar to Polygonum), amenorrhoea and metrorrhagia.

Active Constituents

Have only been recently defined. Potential active constituents include iridoid compounds known as jioglutosides, rehmaglutins, and jioglutins.[1] It also contains other glycosides (jionosides A_1, B_1, C, D).[2,3]

Jioglutoside A

Jionoside A^1

gal = β–D–galactopyranose

Pharmacology

→ Adrenal Cortex Function

- Uncured Rehmannia antagonised the inhibitory action of corticosteroids on plasma corticosterone and inhibited the catabolism of cortisol.[4,5]

→ Immunologic Function

- Constituents in Cured Rehmannia suppressed antibody formation. The immunosuppressive principles of Rehmannia were found to be jionoside A_1, jionoside B_1, acetoside, isoacetoside, purpureaside C, cistanoside A and cistanoside F_2.

- Cured Rehmannia abolished the suppressive effects of cyclophosphamide and dexamethasone on immunity.[6]

- Oral administration of a herbal preparation containing Rehmannia demonstrated protective effects on haematopoiesis, immunity, heart, liver and kidney functions during chemotherapy in tumour-bearing mice.[7]

- Wen-Qing-Yin, a herbal preparation containing nine herbs including Rehmannia, *Scutellaria baicalensis* and Paeony inhibited the induction phases of type IV allergic reactions after oral administration to mice. Local graft-versus-host reaction was also inhibited dose-dependently. The authors believe Wen-Qing-Yin may be of use in treating the cellular immunodeficiency of Behcet's syndrome.[8]

→ Other Effects

- Orally administered Uncured Rehmannia demonstrated improvement in haemorheology in arthritic and thrombotic rats.[9]

- An *in vitro* study has found three compounds of Rehmannia (acetylacteoside, jionoside C and jionoside D) demonstrated aldose reductase inhibitory activity.[3]

- The mutagenic potential of Rehmannia was tested with the Ames test and *in vivo*. Uncured Rehmannia showed no mutagenic activity, whereas cured Rehmannia was mutagenic in the *in vivo* mammalian (mice) assay when given by ip injection.[10]

Clinical Studies

- Uncured Rehmannia produced therapeutic effects in rheumatoid arthritis, asthma and urticaria.

- Oral administration of a herbal preparation containing Rehmannia and Astragalus demonstrated therapeutic effects on chronic nephritis. Improvement was observed in 91% of the treatment group compared to 67% in the control group. Further animal studies verified these therapeutic effects. The preparation also demonstrated antiallergy effects and promotion and modulation of immunity.[11]

Actions (of Uncured Rehmannia)

Antipyretic, antihaemorrhagic, anti-inflammatory.

Medicinal Uses (of Uncured Rehmannia)

- To prevent the suppressive effects of corticosteroid drugs on endogenous levels of corticosteroids.
- Inflammatory disorders involving the immune system, e.g. allergies, especially skin rashes and autoimmune disorders.
- Haemorrhages, e.g. haematuria, metrorrhagia.

Dosage

2 to 6 g/day of the dried (uncured) root or 4 to 12 mL/day of the 1:2 fluid extract.

REFERENCES

1   Morota, T et al: *Phytochemistry* **28**, 2385 (1989).
2   Sasaki, H et al: *Planta Medica* **55**, 458 (1989).
3   Nishimura, H et al: *Planta Medica* **56**, 684 (1990).
4   Cha, L L et al: *Chin J Integ Trad West Med* **8**, 223 (1988) in *Abst Chin Med* **2**, 306 (1988).
5   Chang, H M and But P P: *Pharmacology and Applications of Chinese Materia Medica* Vol 1, World Scientific, Singapore (1986).
6   Li, P et al: *Chin J Immunol* **3**, 296, 320 (1987) in *Abst Chin Med* **2**, 293 (1988).
7   Xu, J P: *Chung-Kuo Chung Hsi I Chieh Ho Tsa Chih* **12**, 709, 734 (1992).
8   Koda, A et al: *Int J Immunopharmac* **9**, 289 (1987).
9   Kubo, M et al: *Biol Pharmaceut Bull* **17**, 1282 (1994).
10 Yin, X J et al: *Mutation Research* **260**, 73 (1991).
11 Su, Z Z et al: *Chung-Kuo Chung Hsi I Chieh Ho Tsa Chih* **13**, 259, 269 (1993).

Rheum palmatum

Also known as *R. officinale and R. tanguticum.*

Mandarin	Da Huang
English	Rhubarb Root
Family	Polygonaceae
Part Used	Root and rhizome

Properties

Bitter and cold. Rhubarb drains heat, invigorates blood and breaks up congealed blood. It is anti-inflammatory and detoxicant and is indicated in constipation, abdominal pain, jaundice due to *damp heat* and amenorrhoea due to blood stasis.

Active Constituents

About 3 to 5% anthraquinones, mostly as glycosides. The laxative activity is mainly due to the sennoside content. The root and rhizome also contain plant phenolics and tannins.[1,2]

Pharmacology

➜ *Laxative Action*

- In patients with "asthenic syndrome" laxative doses may be less effective, or even slow down the intestinal movement.[1]

- Extracts from *Rhamnus frangula*, Rhubarb and Senna exhibited a dose-dependent reduction in gastrointestinal passage time. Combining the three extracts resulted in pure addition of the effects. An extract of *Potentilla anserina*, which when given alone lengthens the passage time, antagonizes the laxative effects of the above extracts. This indicates that tannins counter the effect of anthraquinones. As the laxative effects behaved in a purely additive way they were described as "predictable".[3]

➡ *Antidiarrhoeal Action*

- Low doses (less than 0.3g) often result in constipation due to the dominant effect of the tannins at this dose. The tannins may also inhibit activation of the anthraquinones by gut flora.[1]

➡ *Effect on Liver and Gallbladder*

- Rhubarb promoted secretion of bile and increased its content of bilirubin and bile acids.[1]
- Rhubarb is part of a herbal formula used to treat neonatal jaundice in Asia. Rhubarb increased bilirubin glucuronyl transferase activity in rats.[4]
- Rhubarb as a 20% decoction given at 1 mL/kg orally reduced the mortality and hepatic necrosis in rabbits with toxic hepatitis.[5]

➡ *Antibacterial and Antiviral Action*

- Some anthraquinones in Rhubarb have antibacterial activity, which would further justify its use in diarrhoea. Antifungal, antiparasitical and antiviral effects have also been observed.[1]
- The water extract has been found to have an action against herpes simplex and influenza viruses.[6,7]
- Emodin (an anthraquinone in Rhubarb) demonstrated an inhibitory effect on the pathogenicity of *Trichomonas vaginalis* in mice. It cured the intravaginal infection of trichomonads through oral administration.[8]
- Rhubarb demonstrated high activity against *Helicobacter pylori* transferred from chronic atrophic gastritis patients to cell cultures.[9]
- Hot glycerin extract of Rhubarb inactivated the herpes simplex virus type 1 *in vitro*. Extracted antraquinones were directly virucidal to enveloped viruses. Electron microscope examination of anthraquinone-treated herpes simplex virus demonstrated that the envelopes were partially disrupted.[10]

➡ *Anticancer Activity*

- Anthraquinone aglycones are active against a variety of tumours *in vivo*. Rhubarb has inhibited sarcoma, and anthraquinone derivatives are inhibitory against a leukaemia strain in mice. The effect is thought to be due to the inhibition of respiratory enzymes in cancer cells by the anthraquinones.[1,11]

➡ *Haemostatic Action*

- Rhubarb is locally haemostatic, as could be explained by its tannin content. However it also facilitates blood coagulation and this is probably mediated by the anthraquinones.[1] It increased blood viscosity in rabbits.[12]

➜ *Blood Constituents*

- In rats treated with Rhubarb, urea nitrogen and total cholesterol were significantly lowered.

➜ *Possible Anti-inflammatory Action*

- Hot water extract of rhubarb demonstrated inhibition of arachidonic acid metabolism *in vitro* but not *in vivo*.[13]

- Rhubarb inhibited the synthesis of thromboxane A_2, but had no apparent effect on the synthesis of prostacyclin *in vitro*.[14]

- The effects of rhubarb on arachidonic acid metabolism in renal medulla of rabbits were studied *in vitro*. Rhubarb blocked the biosynthesis of renal medulla prostaglandin E_2 and $F_{2\alpha}$ dose-dependently, and inhibited the biosynthesis of prostaglandin A_2 and thromboxane B_2.[15]

➜ *Effect on the Urinary System*

- Rhubarb inhibited the proliferation of renal tubular cells *in vitro* in a dose-dependent manner. Emodin demonstrated similar activity.[16]

- Rhubarb demonstrated beneficial effects on renal hypertrophy and glomerular filtration rate changes at an early stage in experimental diabetic rats. Rhubarb may therefore be useful in the treatment of diabetic nephropathy.[17]

- Three tannins purified from Rhubarb root were tested on rats with chemically-induced renal failure. Two of the tannins increased the renal functional parameters, such as glomerular filtration rate, renal plasma and blood flow. Urea nitrogen and creatinine were significantly decreased. Not all tannins produced this effect and one component aggravated renal function.[18,19]

- Rhubarb demonstrated a therapeutic effect on experimental early renal damage in rats.[20]

➜ *Other Effects*

- Decoction of Rhubarb lowers body temperature in febrile rabbits, an effect thought to be due to a lowering of cerebral PGE levels.[21]

- Irritability and aggressiveness induced in rats was markedly suppressed by administration of Rhubarb and a mild conditioned evasive response was also suppressed.[22]

- Crude extract of Rhubarb and emodin induced a dose-dependent decrease in the mutagenicity of several chemical mutagens. Emodin reduced the mutagenicity by direct inhibition of hepatic microsomal activation.[23]

- Emodin demonstrated mutagenic activity *in vitro* in the presence of NAD(P)H. Emodin was transformed by microsomal enzymes into several metabolites. 2-Hydroxyemodin proved to be the direct mutagen to the test strain.[24]
- Oral doses of Rhubarb increased delayed hypersensitivity (T cell response) and increased lymphocyte proliferation induced by mitogens.[25]
- Rhubarb was effective in the treatment of experimental haemorrhagic pancreatitis. Blood stasis and pancreatic haemorrhage were less evident in the treated group.[26]

Clinical Studies

→ Haemostatic Action

- Rhubarb, 3g twice daily, was as effective as cimetidine in upper GIT bleeding.[27]
- In 29 open clinical studies, 1703 cases of GIT haemorrhage were treated with Rhubarb at mostly 2 to 3g, 3 to 4 times daily. Haemorrhage was controlled in 94.5% of cases in an average of 3 days. Powder is the most effective dosage form.[28]
- Rhubarb is also effective in high doses for haemobilia (blood in the bile ducts), suggesting a remote mode of action.[29]
- 312 cases of gastric and duodenal ulcer bleeding were treated with 3 kinds of Rhubarb in tablet form. Using double-blind assessment all three species produced an efficiency in the range of 90–94%.[30]

→ Chronic Renal Failure

- Rhubarb is an important tool in the treatment of early stages of chronic renal failure (CRF). It lowers blood urea and creatinine, and improves serum levels of amino acids.[31,32]
- Treatment of CRF with Rhubarb and adjuvant drugs alleviates the suffering of patients and improves the quality of their survival. It can be given to all patients except in very severe cases and can also be used as a transitional measure.[33]
- Baoshen Pill, a Rhubarb extract, was evaluated in a controlled clinical trial on haemodialytic patients. The results showed there were no statistically significant differences between the treatment and control group for blood urea nitrogen and creatinine levels. However, serum total cholesterol and LDL cholesterol fell, and HDL cholesterol increased.[34]
- *In vivo* and *in vitro* studies have demonstrated the effectiveness of Rhubarb in preventing the progression of CRF. A clinical trial was conducted to compare the effects of Rhubarb and the drug Captopril. Long term follow up (6–22 months) showed that the progression rate of renal failure was retarded after

treatment. Rhubarb had a better effect than that of Captopril, but the regime of Rhubarb and Captopril was preferred for long-term prevention of CRF progression.[35,36]

➡ *Anticholesterolaemic Action*

- Rhubarb lowered serum cholesterol and triglycerides, the effective rate for cholesterol being 52% of patients.[37]

- A herbal formula consisting of Rhubarb and *Alismatis orientale* was evaluated on 73 senile hyperlipidaemic patients. Serum cholesterol and triglycerides were measured and a total effective rate of 92% was observed.[38]

➡ *Other Conditions*

- Rhubarb was useful in severe hepatitis with hepatic coma (given as an enema).[5]

- Rhubarb has been used to treat acute pancreatitis in conjunction with orthodox medication.[39]

- Rhubarb was superior to orthodox medication in the treatment of acute enteritis and bacillary dysentery.[40]

- There are some reports that Rhubarb may cause remission of malignant tumours.[1]

- A double blind study observed that processed Rhubarb (0.75 g/day) produced a prophylactic effect in pregnant women at risk of pregnancy induced hypertension (PIH). Only 5.7% of the women developed PIH compared to 20.8% in the untreated group.[41] Note: Raw unprocessed Rhubarb root is generally considered to be contraindicated in pregnancy and lactation.

- A Chinese herbal formula with Rhubarb as the main ingredient was tested in an open clinical trial on patients with endometriosis. Endometriotic Pill No 1 yielded distinct improvement in clinical signs and symptoms, and laboratory assay of blood rheology, serum immunoglobulins and prostaglandin.[42]

- In a uncontrolled study, the topical application of a combination of Rhubarb alcoholic extract and salicylic acid was studied in 95 cases involving lesions of the buccal mucosa. Good results were obtained for the treatment of cases of oral inflammation and ulceration, including gum disease. Analgesic, anti-inflammatory and healing actions were noted for the preparation.[43]

 ## Actions

Laxative, haemostatic, antipyretic, antibacterial, astringent, anti-inflammatory, antiuraemic.

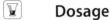

Medicinal Uses

- Constipation, enteritis, dysentery, gastrointestinal haemorrhage.
- Acute hepatitis and pancreatitis in conjunction with other agents.
- Early stages of chronic renal failure in conjunction with other agents.
- Fevers.
- Hyperlipidaemia in conjunction with other treatments.
- May be useful in acute cholecystitis and cancer.

Dosage

1 to 6 g/day of the dried root/rhizome or 2 to 12 mL/day of the 1:2 fluid extract.

REFERENCES

1   Chang, H M and But P P: *Pharmacology and Applications of Chinese Materia Medica*, Vol, World Scientific, Singapore (1987).

2   Tang, W and Eisenbrand, G: *Chinese Drugs of Plant Origin*, Springer Verlag, Berlin (1992).

3   Vogel, G: *Arzneim-Forsch* **25**, 1356 (1975).

4   Yin, J et al: *Devel Pharmacol Therapeut* **20**, 186 (1993).

5   Hu, L H et al: *Chin J Integ Trad West Med* **6**, 41 (1986) in *Abst Chin Med* **1**, 440 (1987).

6   May, G et al: *Arzneim-Forsch* **28**, 1 (1978) in *Kampo TCM Update* Chinaherb Co P/L Redfern **2**, 7 (1995).

7   Chen, Q H et al: *J Trad Chin Med* **5**, 34 (1974) *Kampo TCM Update* Chinaherb Co P/L Redfern **2**, 7 (1995).

8   Wang, H H: *J Ethnopharmacol* **40**, 111 (1993).

9   Zhang, L et al: *Chung Kuo Chung Hsi I Chieh Ho Tsa Chih* **12**, 515, 521 (1992).

10   Sydiskis, R J et al: *Antimicrob Agents Chemother* **35**, 2463 (1991).

11   Lu, M and Chen, Q H: *J China Pharm Univ* **20**, 155 (1989) *Kampo TCM Update* Chinaherb Co P/L Redfern **2**, 7 (1995).

12   Liang, Z J et al: *Chin J Integ Trad West Med* **6**, 294 (1986) in *Abst Chin Med* **1**, 384 (1987).

13   Umeda, M et al: *J Ethnopharmacol* **23**, 91 (1988).

14   Wang, S R et al: *Chung Kuo Chung Hsi I Chieh Ho Tsa Chih* **13**, 134, 167 (1993).

15   Guo, C Y et al: *Chung Hsi I Chieh Ho Tsa Chih* **9**, 161, 134 (1989).

16   Zheng, F: *Chung-Hsa I Hsueh Tsa Chih* **73**, 343, 380 (1993).

17   Yang, J W and Li, L S: *Chung Kuo Chung Hsi I Chieh Ho Tsa Chih* **13**, 261, 286 (1993).

18   Yokozawa, T et al: *Nippon Jinzo Gakkai Shi* **35**, 13 (1993).

19   Yokozawa, T et al: *Nephron* **58**, 155 (1991).

20   Luo, J A et al: *Chung Kuo Chung Hsi I Chieh Ho Tsa Chih* **13**, 70, 98 (1993).

21   Guo, C Y et al: *Chin J Integ Trad West Med* **6**, 109 (1986) in *Abst Chin Med* **1**, 383 (1987).

22   Nokia, A: *Gen Dai To Yo I Gaku* **7**, 98 (1986) *Kampo TCM Update* Chinaherb Co P/L Redfern **2**, 7 (1995).

23   Lee H and Tsai, S J: *Food Chem Toxicol* **29**, 765 (1991).

24   Masuda, T and Ueno, T: *Mutation Res* **125**, 135 (1984).

25   Ma, L: *Chung Kuo Chung Hsi I Chieh Ho Tsa Chih* **11**, 390, 418 (1991).

26   Ren, S: *Chung Hsi I Chieh Ho Tsa Chih* **10**, 133, 162 (1990).

27   Sun, D A et al: *Chin J Integ Trad West Med* **6**, 458 (1986) in *Abst Chin Med* **1**, 431 (1987).

28   Jiao, D H et al: *Zhongchengyao Yanjiu* p21, (1987) in *Abst Chin Med* **2**, 231 (1988).

29   Jin, Q F et al: *Shanghai J Trad Chin Med* p5, (1988) in *Abst Chin Med* **3**, 72 (1989).

30   Zhou, H and Jiao, D: *Chung Hsi I Chieh Ho Tsa Chih* **10**, 131, 150 (1990).

31   Song, C: *J Shandong Col Trad Chin Med* **13**, 204 (1989) in *Abst Chin Med* **3**, 211 (1989).

32   Yang, R Z et al: *Chin J Nephrol* **5**, 247 (1989) in *Abst Chin Med* **3**, 161 (1989).

33   Kang, Z et al: *J Trad Chin Med* **13**, 249 (1993).

34   Ji, S M et al: *Chung Kuo Chung Hsi I Chieh Ho Tsa Chih* **13**, 67, 71 (1993).

35   Li, L S and Liu, Z H: *Chung Hsi I Chieh Ho Tsa Chih* **11**, 387, 392 (1991).

36   Zhang, J H et al: *Chin Med J* **103**, 788 (1990).

37   Jiao, D H et al: *Shanghai J Trad Chin Med* p2, (1988) in *Abst Chin Med* **3**, 58 (1989).

38   Xu, F and Fu, H M: *Chung Kuo Chung Hsi I Chieh Ho Tsa Chih* **13**, 643, 655 (1993).

39   Xia, X D et al: *Jiangxi J Trad Chin Med Pharmacol* **19**, 19 (1988) in *Abst Chin Med* **2**, 445 (1988).

40   Qian, S T et al: *Chin Trad Patent Med* **11**, 23 (1989) in *Abst Chin Med* **3**, 382 (1989).

41   Zhang, Z T et al: *Chin J Obs Gyn* (Engl) **29**, 463, 509 (1994).

42   Wang, D Z et al: *Chung Hsi I Chieh Ho Tsa Chih* **11**, 515, 524 (1991).

43   Pons, J and Bouhours, G: *Information Dentaire* **53**, 3201 (1971).

Salvia miltiorrhiza

Mandarin	Dan Shen
English	Red Root Sage
Family	Lamiaceae
Part Used	Root

Properties

Bitter and slightly cold. Dan Shen a blood stimulant and blood stasis remover with sedative action. It is used in angina, insomnia, palpitations, menstrual problems, impact injuries and liver disease.[1]

Active Constituents

A series of diterpene diketones known as tanshinones: tanshinones 1, 2A and 2B, cryptotanshinone, isotanshinones 1 and 2 etc.[1] Tanshinone 2A is the main constituent which may be up to 0.5%.[2]

Water soluble tanshinone II sodium sulfonate

Pharmacology

→ *Cardiovascular System*

MYOCARDIAL ISCHAEMIA

- Dan Shen improved coronary blood flow *in vivo* and in isolated heart preparations.[1]
- ECG abnormalities due to myocardial ischaemia *in vivo* could be counteracted.[1] Ischaemic damage was decreased and recovery was accelerated and this was confirmed in microscopical studies.[1]
- Collateral coronary circulation is activated thereby improving blood flow into the ischaemic area of the heart.[1]
- Tanshinone 2A is comparable to verapamil in reducing Ca uptake by myocardium.[3]
- Dan Shen prevents the drop in myocardial ATP induced by ischaemia.[4]
- Oral administration of tanshinone to rabbits with experimental myocardial infarction suppressed neutrophil function dose-dependently and concomitantly reduced myocardial necrosis.[5]
- Intraperitoneal injection of water extract of Dan Shen to rats can prevent acute myocardial ischaemia induced by ligation. In the treated group the ischaemic area in the left ventricle was reduced and survival rate increased.[6]
- Tanshinone VI water-soluble derivatives improved post-hypoxic contractile recovery from hypoxic isolated rat hearts.[7]
- Tanshindiol B elicited significant recovery of contractile force upon reoxygenation using isolated, perfused rat hearts.[8]

BLOOD PRESSURE

- Dan Shen has a mild vasodilatory action which causes a drop in blood pressure.[1]

CARDIAC OUTPUT

- Dan Shen is not cardiotonic and does not increase cardiac output, although it potentiates the effect of other cardiotonic herbs e.g. Astragalus.[9]

EFFECTS ON PLATELET FUNCTION AND COAGULATION

- Dan Shen is a potent inhibitor of platelet activity and this is mainly due to the minor tanshinone derivatives in the root.[1,10]
- Thrombosis time is prolonged and thrombus size is reduced.[1]
- *In vitro* experiments have demonstrated anticoagulant and fibrinolytic activities for Dan Shen.[1]

EFFECTS ON MICROCIRCULATION

- In rabbits with peripheral circulatory disturbances, Dan Shen could significantly improve blood flow in the microcirculation and deaggregate red blood cells.[1]

OTHER EFFECTS

- *In vitro* studies on the viscoelastic properties of red cell suspensions suggest that Dan Shen could improve the viscoelastic properties of whole blood.[11]

- Aqueous extract of Dan Shen demonstrated endothelium-dependent vasodilation *in vitro*. The active component was found to be lithospermic acid.[12]

- The effect of intraperitoneal injection of Dan Shen on warfarin was investigated in rats. Dan Shen increased the initial bioavailability of warfarin and affected its elimination. Dan Shen further increases the prothrombin time after warfarin treatment.[13]

- Intravenous pretreatment with aqueous extract of Dan Shen raised the survival rate of rats with chemically-induced ventricular fibrillation.[14]

➜ *Hepatoprotective Effects*

- Dan Shen protects against carbon tetrachloride liver injury and experimental cirrhosis, and prevents hepatic fibrosis.[15]

- It causes increased RNA and protein synthesis in isolated hepatocytes.[16]

- Dan Shen and *Paeonia lactiflora* demonstrated a protective effect in experimental liver damage.[17]

➜ *Antioxidant Effects*

- Treatment with SOD (a free radical scavenger) and Dan Shen prior to the onset of reperfusion protected epigastric island skin flaps in rats, indicating a reduction in ischaemia-reperfusion injury.[18]

- Antioxidants such as vitamin E and Dan Shen exhibited protective effects against multiple organ injuries through a free radical scavenging mechanism.[19]

- Three water-soluble components of Dan Shen demonstrated strong inhibition of chemically-induced lipid peroxidation *in vitro*. The antioxidant activity may be due to scavenging the O^{2-} radical.[20]

- Seven phenolic compounds from Dan Shen inhibited peroxidation of rat liver microsomes and inhibited chemically-induced haemolysis of rat erythrocytes. Salvianolic acid A demonstrated the most potent activity.[21]

➜ *Healing of Fractures*

- Dan Shen causes early formation of dense callus in rabbits with experimental fracture. Microscopic examination revealed increased activity of osteoblasts, fibroblasts etc.[22]

➜ *Pulmonary Fibrosis*

- A potent component isolated from Dan Shen demonstrated prophylactic and therapeutic effects on pulmonary fibrosis in rats.[23]

- In an earlier study the component exerted a direct inhibitory effect on fibroblast proliferation and decreased their ability to synthesize collagen.[24]

➜ *Renal Protective*

- Dan Shen partially protects renal function and structure against chemical and ischaemic damage.[25]

➜ *Hypoxia Tolerance*

- Survival under conditions of hypoxia is prolonged by both Dan Shen and tan-shinone 2A.[1]

➜ *Immunologic Function and Cytoxic Effects*

- A water soluble component extracted from Dan Shen was able to promote macrophage synthesis of the C4 component of complement *in vitro* and *in vivo*.[26]

- Ether and hot water extracts of Dan Shen root enhanced the activity of two mutagens at low concentrations, but suppressed them at high concentrations.[27]

- Several tanshinones demonstrated cytotoxic activity against human carcinoma cell lines *in vitro*.[28]

➜ *Other Effects*

- Dan Shen has mild sedative and antibacterial effects and may lower blood lipids.[1]

- Dan Shen demonstrated a number of effects on the endocrine function of ovaries in rats. Dan Shen increased the level of estradiol in plasma, the weight of uterus and ovarian $PGF_{2\alpha}$ content. It also stimulated ovulation in immature mice pretreated with animal gonadotropin. In pseudopregnant rats it inhibited the function of corpus luteum and decreased the level of plasma progesterone.[29]

- Miltirone, a diterpene isolated from Dan Shen behaved as a partial agonist in the central benzodiazapine receptor binding and behavioural tests. It produced no acute muscle relaxant effect and did not induce drug dependence and withdrawal reactions after chronic administration.[30]

- Investigation into the structure-activity relationship of miltirone suggest that its ring A is essential for binding affinity to the central benzodiazepine receptor.[31]

Clinical Studies

→ *Cardiovascular Conditions*

- More than 300 heart patients were treated with oral doses of Dan Shen in an open study. Angina was improved in 81% and abnormal ECG in 57%.[1]

- Dan Shen injection is used to treat acute heart attacks in Chinese hospitals. Mortality rate fell from 39% to 13%. Early application within 24 hours of the attack is necessary.[32]

- Dan Shen is part of a formula which has been used in other Chinese hospitals to significantly lower mortality from heart attacks.[33]

- Dan Shen injection lowered BP in hypertensive patients.[1]

- Dan Shen injection improved recovery from stroke (although caution should be exercised so that BP is not lowered too rapidly).[1]

- The effect of nitroglycerin and Dan Shen were compared in 20 patients with ischaemic heart disease. Dan Shen was markedly superior to nitroglycerin, with more persistent effects and also improved cardiac function.[34]

- An open clinical trial found treatment combining Dan Shen intravenous drip with heparin vapour inhalation to be an efficient therapy for anticoagulation in patients with pulmonary heart disease.[35]

- Dan Shen injection gave good results in disseminated intravascular coagulation.[1]

- Positive results were obtained in Buerger's disease.[1]

- In a controlled clinical trial, Dan Shen was found to reduce lipid peroxide reaction, adjust the imbalance of antioxidant enzymes and enhance the body's defence capability against free radical induced lipid peroxidation.[36]

- In a group of 20 patients with hyperviscosity syndrome treated with an aqueous extract of Dan Shen, serum levels of the C4 component of complement rose, which correlated with the disappearance of clinical symptoms.[26]

→ *Hepatitis*

- Satisfactory results were obtained for chronic hepatitis, and for acute hepatitis in combination with *Hypericum japonicum*.[1]

- Combined with Turmeric and *Crataegus pinnatifida*, a 69% cure rate was obtained in chronic active hepatitis.[37]

➡ *Other Conditions*

- Tanshinones at high doses over eight weeks markedly improved acne in more than 50% of cases.[38]

- Dan Shen injection gave good results in nerve compression syndromes and with Rehmannia gave significant improvement in diabetic neuropathy.[39,40]

- For lymphoma, Dan Shen in combination with chemotherapy was significantly better than just chemotherapy.[41]

Actions

Cardioprotective, hypotensive, anticoagulant, antiplatelet, fibrinolytic, hepatoprotective, vulnerary, antifibrotic, antibacterial.

Medicinal Uses

- Ischaemic heart disease (angina, heart attacks etc).
- High blood pressure.
- Palpitations.
- Impaired peripheral and cerebrovascular circulation, Buerger's disease.
- Acute and chronic liver disease.
- Promotion of healing of fractures and other injuries.
- Scleroderma and other autoimmune disorders.
- Pulmonary fibrosis.
- Nerve compression and diabetic neuropathy.
- Acne and other skin disorders.
- As an adjunct to treatment of lymphoma.

Contraindications

- Anticoagulant and antiplatelet drugs.
- Bleeding tendency.
- Pregnancy.

Dosage

2 to 6 g/day of the dried root or 4 to 12 mL/day of 1:2 fluid extract.

REFERENCES

1   Chang, H and But, P: *Pharmacology and Applications of Chinese Materia Medica*, Vol 1, World Scientific, Singapore (1986).

2   Zheng, G C et al: *Chin Pharmaceut J* **24**, 6 (1989) in *Abst Chin Med* **3**, 81 (1989).

3   Yue, P et al: *Chin J Pathophysiol* **3**, 154 (1987) in *Abst Chin Med* **2**, 316 (1988).

4   Ma, L et al: *Chin J Pathophys* **4**, 84 (1988).

5   Li, X H and Tang, R Y: *Chung-Kuo Yao Li Hsueh Pao* **12**, 269 (1991).

6   Cheng, Y Y et al: *Chung-Kuo Chung Hsi i Chieh Ho Tsa Chih* **12**, 424 (1992).

7   Yagi, A et al: *Planta Medica* **60**, 405 (1994).

8   Yagi, A et al: *Planta Medica* **57**, 228 (1991).

9   Zhu, B et al: *Chin J Integ Trad Western Med* **7**, 591 (1987).

10   Wang, N et al: *Plant Medica* **55**, 390 (1989).

11   Yang, Y: *Hua Hsi i Ko Ta Hsueh Hsueh Pao* **24**, 143 (1993).

12   Kamata, K: *General Pharmacol* **24**, 977 (1993).

13   Lo, A C et al: *Eur J Drug Metab Pharmacokin* **17**, 257 (1992).

14   Cheng, Y Y et al: *Chung Hsi i Chieh Ho Tsa Chih* **11**, 518, 543 (1991).

15   Ma, X H et al: *Chin J Integ Trad Western Med* **8**, 161 (1988) in *Abst Chin Med* **2**, 312 (1988).

16   Xu, C H et al: *Bull Chin Materia Medica* **13**, 557 (1988) in *Abst Chin Med* **3**, 42 (1989).

17   Qi, X G: *Chung Hsi i Chieh Ho Tsa Chih* **11**, 69, 102 (1991).

18   Yang, D P: *Chung-Hua Cheng Hsing Shao Shang Wai Ko Tsa Chih* **8**, 216 (1992).

19   Fu, X et al: *Chin Med Sc J* **7**, 86 (1992).

20   Huang, Y S and Zhang J J: *Yao Hsueh Hsueh Pao* **27**, 96 (1992).

21   Liu, G T: *Biochem Pharmacol* **43**, 147 (1992).

22   Chai, B F et al: *Chin J Integ Trad Western Med* **7**, 417 (1987) in *Abst Chin Med* **2**, 156 (1988).

23   Liu, J et al: *Chin Med Sc J* **8**, 9 (1993).

24   Liu, J et al: *Chin Med Sc J* **7**, 142 (1992).

25   Shen, Y C et al: *Chin J Exp Surg* **5**, 23 (1988) in *Abst Chin Med* **2**, 312 (1988).

26   Ling M et al: *Exp Clin Immunogenetics* **10**, 45 (1993).

27   Sato, M et al: *Mutation Research* **265**, 149 (1992).

28   Wu, W L et al: *Am J Chin Med* **19**, 207 (1991).

29   Li, W et al: *Chung-Kuo Chung Hsi i Chieh Ho Tsa Chih* **12**, 165 (1992).

30   Lee, C M et al: *Neuroscience Letters* **127**, 237 (1991).

31   Chang, H M et al: *J Med Chem* **34**, 1675 (1991).

32   Keji, C: *Am J Chin Med* **9**, 193 (1981).

33   Guo, S K et al: *Plant Medica* **48**, 63 (1983).

34   Bai, Y R and Wang, S Z: *Chung-Kuo Chung Hsi i Chieh Ho Tsa Chih* **14**, 4, 24 (1994).

35   Zhang, F C and Zheng, L J: *Chung Hsi i Chieh Ho Tsa Chih* **11**, 579, 589 (1991).

36   Zhang, P T and Chen, Z R: *Chung-Kuo Chung Hsi i Chien Ho Tsa Chih* **14**, 474 (1994).

37   Liao, K Y et al: *Sichuanzhongui* **5**, 18 (1987) in *Abst Chin Med* **2**, 336 (1988).

38   Wang, D B et al: *Chin J Dermatol* **21**, 167 (1988) in *Abst Chin Med* **3**, 56 (1989).

39   Bi, X L et al: *Chin J Integ Trad Western Med* **8**, 84 (1988) in *Abst Chin Med* **2**, 341 (1988).

40   Yang, Z L and Hou B X: *Shanghai J Trad Chin Med* **2**, 28 (1987) in *Abst Chin Med* **2**, 58 (1988).

41   Zhang, Y W et al: *J Xi'an Medical Uni* **10**, 180 (1989) in *Abst Chin Med* **3**, 202 (1989).

Schisandra chinensis

Mandarin	Wu Wei Zi
English	Schisandra Fruit, Chinese Magnolia Vine
Family	Schisandraceae
Part Used	Fruit

Properties

Sour and warm. Schisandra is reputed to be "kidney"-tonifying and sedative. It is mainly used to treat cough and wheezing, spontaneous sweating, nocturnal emission, chronic diarrhoea, insomnia and forgetfulness.[1] In Russia it is regarded as an adaptogen.

Active Constituents

A large number of dibenzocyclooctane lignans known as schizandrins and gomisins.[2] Also triterpenic acids, triterpenic lactones, essential oil, citric acid, and vitamins C and E.[1]

Schisandrin

Gomisin D

⁖ Pharmacology

➜ *Hepatoprotective Effects and Effects on Hepatic Metabolism*

- Schisandra and its lignans reduce the enzymatic and morphological changes indicative of liver damage following many liver toxins.[3]

- Schisandra lignans stimulate liver glycogen synthesis, protein synthesis and elevate liver microsomal drug-metabolising enzyme activities.[3]

- The observed protective action against carbon tetrachloride hepatotoxicity may be due to the inhibitory effects on lipid-peroxidation.[3]

- Schisandra lignans increase microsomal cytochrome P-450 concentrations and also other detoxifying enzymes. However, Schisandra lignans do not increase benzopyrene mutagenicity — it is in fact decreased.[3]

- Another study found that a lignan component of Schisandra stimulated liver regeneration after partial hepatectomy in rats. Ornithine decarboxylase activity, an important biochemical event in the early stages of liver regeneration, was enhanced.[4]

- Gomisin A protected the liver of rats from injury after administration of acetaminophen through the suppression of lipid peroxidation.[5]

- Seven lignans isolated from Schisandraceae demonstrated antioxidant activity in rat liver *in vitro*. The action was more potent than vitamin E at the same concentration. Schisanhenol, the most active lignan, prevented the decrease of membrane fluidity of liver microsomes induced by chemicals.[6]

- Schisandrin B was shown to maintain the membrane stability of rat hepatocytes *in vitro* under oxidative stress.[7]

- A synthetic schisandrin derivative called DDB is widely used in China as a hepatoprotective drug, with high effectiveness in normalizing liver functions and very few side effects.[8]

- Schisandra lignans increased survival in experimental acute fulminant hepatitis from 7.5 to 80% and prevented liver cell necrosis.[3]

- Schisandra was shown to inhibit the reductive metabolism of an anaesthetic halothane *in vitro*. Schisandra may protect against halothane-induced hepatitis.[9]

- One study has shown that Schisandra decreases transaminase in the liver which may indicate a decreased detoxicant ability, which exposes the liver to damage.[1]

- Gomisin A improved the survival rate and serum transaminase levels of immunologically-induced acute hepatic failure guinea pigs. Histological changes in the liver were also improved.[10] Further work indicated that oral administration of gomisin A may prevent the development of immunologically-induced acute hepatic failure.[11]

➜ *Mental Performance*

• Although the lignans have a depressive effect on the CNS,[12] the total extract has a stimulant effect.[1]

• Injection of schisandrol A to rats resulted in inhibition of the CNS. The inhibition may be related to the dopamine system. The metabolism of noradrenaline and serotonin were affected, but their concentrations were unchanged.[13]

• Schisandra exhibits antidepressant activity in mice.[14]

• Learning ability of mice is improved.[15]

➜ *Adaptogenic and Tonic Effects*

• Schisandra increases human endurance.[15]

• Schisandra increased RNA, glycogen and enzymes in kidneys and gonads of mature rabbits, returning these values to those of three month-old rabbits. It also increased the number of reproductive cells in males and females.[16]

➜ *Cancer Prevention*

• Gomisin A demonstrated a strong inhibitory effect on skin tumour promotion in mice. The effect is believed to be due to its anti-inflammatory activity.[17]

• Oral administration of gomisin A by showed a weak suppressive effect on tumour promotion in the liver of rats.[18]

• Gomisin A demonstrated an inhibitory effect on hepatocarcinogenesis in rats. The effect is likely to be related to improved liver function and reversal of abnormal cell multiplication. An earlier study indicated gomisin A enhanced the excretion of carcinogens from the liver and reversed the cytokinesis.[20]

➜ *Other Effects*

• Lignans decrease cardiac but not skeletal muscle necrosis in dystrophic hamsters.[21]

• Schisandra stimulates respiration and has expectorant and antitussive effects.[1]

• Schisandra stimulates uterine contraction.[1]

• Schisanhenol and schisandrin B have a protective action against oxidative stress in rat brain *in vitro*. Schisanhenol demonstrated stronger activity and other studies have confirmed its potent antioxidant activities.[22,23]

• Gomisin C inhibited the respiratory burst of rat neutrophils *in vitro*. This action was not mediated by changes in cellular cAMP or by oxygen free radical scavengers released from neutrophils.[24]

- Schisanhenol demonstrated protection against adriamycin toxicity in rat heart mitochondria[25] but did not antagonize the anti-tumour activity of adriamycin.[26]

Pharmacokinetics

- *In vitro* and *in vivo* studies indicate that schisandrin is metabolized to several compounds including 7,8-dihydroxy-schisandrin and two 7,8-dihydroxy-dimethylschisandrins in rat liver.[27]
- Gomisin A undergoes a first pass effect and is transformed into its major metabolites rapidly after both intravenous and oral administration.[28]
- In carbon tetrachloride-treated rats, the body clearance of gomisin A decreased to less than half that in normal rats, even when administered orally.[29]
- Oral administration of 10 mg/kg of gomisin A to rats resulted in a maximum serum concentration of approximately 1400 ng/mL and 300 ng/mL of its metabolite.[30]

Clinical Studies

- In many open clinical studies the herb significantly reduced elevated serum glutamic-pyruvic transaminase (SGPT) levels in various types of hepatitis. However SGPT levels rebounded after stopping the herb, especially in chronic persistent hepatitis.[1]
- One theory is that the herb inhibits enzyme synthesis in damaged liver cells, and therefore reduction of SGPT is not correlated with clinical improvement.[1] However this is not consistent with much of the pharmacological studies.
- In one controlled trial in chronic viral hepatitis, SGPT levels were normalised and no rebound was observed. Improvement of other liver function tests were less pronounced.[3]
- Small open clinical studies have shown benefit in induction of labour, mild spastic paralysis following a stroke, Parkinson's disease, cerebellar ataxia, Ménière syndrome and psychosis.[1]
- Schisandra improved mental efficiency, sensitivity of sight and hearing, increased the speed of adaptation to the dark, enlarged the visual field and increased the discrimination of skin receptors.[1]
- The lignans improve activities requiring concentration and fine co-ordination in humans.[1]

Actions

Hepatoprotective, nervine tonic, adaptogenic, antitussive.

Medicinal Uses

- Acute and chronic liver diseases, in conjunction with other herbs.
- Chemical liver damage, poor liver function.
- To improve the detoxifying capacity of the liver.
- To improve mental, physical and sensory performance.
- Nervous system disorders.
- Contraindicated in pregnancy except to facilitate childbirth.

Dosage

1.5 to 6 g/day of the dried fruit, 3 to 12 mL/day of 1:2 fluid extract.

REFERENCES

1   Chang, H M and But, P P: *Pharmacology and Applications of Chinese Materia Medica* Vol 1, World Scientific, Singapore (1987).

2   Tang, W and Eisenbrand, G: *Chinese Drugs of Plant Origin*, Springer Verlag, Berlin (1992).

3   Hikino, H and Kiso, Y: *Natural Products for Liver Diseases* in Wagner H et al, (eds) *Economic and Medicinal Plant Research,* Vol 2, Academic Press (1988).

4   Kubo, S: *Planta Medica* **58**, 489 (1992).

5   Yamada, S et al: *Biochem Pharmacol* **46**, 1081 (1993).

6   Lu, H and Liu, G T: *Planta Medica* **58**, 311 (1992).

7   Zhang, T M et al: *Chung-Kuo Yao Li Hsueh Pao* **13**, 255 (1992).

8   Li, X Y: *Memorias do Instituto Oswaldo Cruz* **86**, 31 (1991).

9   Jiaxiang N et al: *J Appl Toxicol* **13**, 385 (1993).

10 Mizoguchi Y et al: *Planta Medica* **57**, 11 (1991).

11 Mizoguchi Y et al: *Planta Medica* **57**, 320 (1991).

12 Li, L N: *Abst Chin Med* **3**, 414 (1989).

13 Zhang, L and Niu, X: *Chung-Kuo i Hsueh Ko Hsueh Yuan Hsueh Pao* **13**, 13 (1991).

14 Hancke, J L et al: *Planta Medica* **52**, 542 (1986).

15 Fulder, S: *The Root of Being,* Hutchinson and Co, London (1980).

16 Peng G R et al: *Shanghai J Trad Chin Med* p43 (1989) in *Abst Chin Med* **3**, 157 (1989).

17 Yasukawa, K et al: *Oncology* **49**, 68 (1992).

18 Miyamoto K et al: *Jap J Pharmacol* **57**, 71 (1991).

19 Nomura M et al: *Anticancer Res* **14**, 1967 (1994).

20 Ohtaki, Y et al: *Biol Pharmaceut Bull* **17**, 808 (1994).

21 Shen, D G et al: *Muscle and Nerve* **10**, 391 (1987).

22 Xue, J Y et al: *Free Radical Biol Med* **12**, 127 (1992).

23 Lin T J et al: *Biomed Environ Sci* **5**, 57 (1992).

24 Wang, J P et al: *Brit J Pharmacol* **113**, 945 (1994).

25 Lin T J et al: *Biochem Pharmacol* **42**, 1805 (1991).

26 Lin T J and Liu G T: *Biochem Biophys Res Commun* **178**, 207 (1991).

27 Cui, Y Y and Wang, M Z: *Eur J Drug Metab Pharmacokin* **18**, 155 (1993).

28   Matsuzaki Y et al: *Yakugaku Zasshi* **111**, 524 (1991).

29   Matsuzaki Y et al: *Yakugaku Zasshi* **111**, 531 (1991).

30   Matsuzaki Y et al: *Yakugaku Zasshi* **111**, 617 (1991).

Scutellaria baicalensis

Mandarin	Huang Qin
English	Baikal (or Baical) Skullcap Root, Scute
Family	Lamiaceae
Part Used	Root

Properties

Bitter and cold. Clears heat and damp heat. Also used for abnormal foetal movements and for allergic and inflammatory diseases.[1]

Active Constituents

Mainly flavones and flavone glycosides such as baicalein, baicalin and wogonin. Baicalin is the major component and estimates vary from 12–17% to 6.4–9.9% of the weight of the dried root.[2,3] Baicalin can undergo decomposition to its aglycone which is baicalein (0.5%).[2]

	R
Baicalin	D-glucuronic acid
Baicalein	H

	R
Wogonoside	D-glucuronic acid
Wogonin	H

Pharmacology

→ Antiallergic and Anti-inflammatory Effects

- Flavonoids are known to inhibit prostaglandin production and histamine release by mast cells *in vitro*,[4] and also binding between antigens and IgE.[5]

- Both baicalin and baicalein inhibit antigen-induced allergic contraction in the lungs of sensitised animals and anaphylaxis in animal models. The aglycone is stronger in effect.[6]
- Flavonoids of Baikal Skullcap are strong inhibitors of lipoxygenase and cyclooxygenase in vitro, with aglycones being stronger in effect.[7]
- Baikal Skullcap inhibits the production of prostaglandins and leukotrienes. Baicalein inhibited the biosynthesis of leukotrienes B_4 and C_4 in human leukocytes.[8,9]
- Baicalein showed strong anti-inflammatory activity in a chronic inflammation model (rat adjuvant arthritis).[10]
- Baikal Skullcap flavonoids demonstrated anti-inflammatory activity similar to that of prednisolone in vitro.[11]
- Direct addition of hot water extract of Baikal Skullcap to a selected enzyme medium inhibited arachidonic acid (AA) biotransformation. The serum of rats orally pretreated for 1 hour with Baikal Skullcap root did not however inhibit AA biotransformation.[12]

➡ **Potential Antiplatelet Effects**

- Baicalein, wogonin and other flavonoids inhibited collagen- and arachidonic acid-induced platelet aggregation.[13]

➡ **Antioxidant Effects**

- Skullcap flavonoids inhibit lipid peroxidation in rat liver in vitro.[14] Baicalein also acted as a free radical scavenger.[15]
- Baikal Skullcap extract was found to exert significant antioxidant activity in several tests.[16] Baicalein quenched superoxide and hydroxyl free radicals in a dose-dependent manner and demonstrated antiepileptic and neuronal protective effects.[17]

➡ **Phosphodiesterase Inhibition**

- The crude extract inhibits phosphodiesterase. This raises cAMP and results in antiplatelet and hypotensive effects (vasodilation).[5]
- The hypotensive effect has been confirmed many times in animal experiments.[2]

➡ **Diuretic Effect**

- Whole extracts or individual flavonoids produce diuresis when given orally or by injection. This effect is thought to be mediated by prostaglandins.[2]

➜ *Aldose Reductase Inhibition*

- Skullcap flavonoids are potent inhibitors of aldose reductase *in vitro* and *in vivo*.[5]

➜ *Antimicrobial and Antiviral Action*

- The antimicrobial action is probably due to the flavonoids (analogous to Propolis) and is demonstrated against a broad spectrum of organisms.[3,6]
- Baicalin was found to inhibit HIV-1 infection and replication *in vitro*.[18]

➜ *Cytotoxic and Antitumour Action*

- *In vitro* studies have found Skullcap flavone II is cytotoxic against mouse leukemia cells.[19]
- Baicalin exhibits antitumour effects against human hepatoma cells.[20]
- Baicalein exhibited an antiproliferative activity in human T-lymphoid leukemia cells. Baicalein may affect cell proliferation by direct inhibition of growth-related enzymes, and in particular platelet-derived growth factor.[21]
- Baicalein was more effective than baicalin and wogonin in inhibiting smooth muscle cell proliferation *in vitro*.[22]

➜ *Inhibition of Lipogenesis*

- Lipogenesis in hamster sebaceous glands was suppressed 54% by wogonin *in vitro*. Baikal Skullcap may therefore be useful in the topical treatment of acne vulgaris.[23]

➜ *Potential Anticoagulant Activity*

- An *in vitro* study found baicalein to be a new type of inhibitor of the vitamin K reductase group of enzymes with potential as an oral anticoagulant drug. Results indicate that baicalein binds to different sites than those of dicoumarol.[24] However, this activity has not been confirmed *in vivo*.

➜ *Kidney Function*

- In an *in vitro* study, baicalein inhibited angiotensin II-induced increases in the cellular protein content of aortic smooth muscle cells.[25] Baicalein also attenuated the angiotensin II-induced increase in renal vascular resistance by approximately 50% and promoted an increase in glomerular filtration rate *in vitro*.[26]
- Pretreatment of rats with baicalein significantly inhibited the decrease in glomerular filtration rate and renal blood flow following administration of a nephrotoxin.[27]

→ *Other Effects*

- Baikal Skullcap flavonoids also enhanced cellular activity in gingival fibroblasts. Hence Baikal Skullcap extract may have therapeutic application in periodontal disease.[11]

Pharmacokinetics

- Most flavonoid glycosides (such as baicalin) pass through the gut unchanged until they reach the large intestine where they are converted into the aglycone by bacterial action. The aglycone is therefore the active form (baicalein and wogonin). Despite this, baicalein has demonstrated lower bioavailability than baicalin possibly due to its poor water solubility. *In vitro* studies of flavonoid glycosides may have little clinical relevance except for topical use or administration by injection.[28,29,30]

Clinical Studies

→ *Infections*

- Positive results have been shown for the following infections — acute bronchitis, colds, bacillary dysentery, scarlet fever, hepatitis and cholecystitis. These were open studies with no placebo controls.[2]

→ *Hypertension*

- An antihypertensive effect was demonstrated in an open study of 51 cases.[2]

→ *Chronic Hepatitis*

- A 70% success rate has been shown in chronic hepatitis with improvements in symptoms and liver function tests.

→ *Allergic Rhinitis*

- Baikal Skullcap was successfully used in combination with other herbs for the treatment of this disorder.[31]

Actions

Anti-inflammatory, antiallergic, antibacterial, mild sedative, hypotensive, diuretic, bitter.

Medicinal Uses

- Allergic conditions such as hayfever, asthma, urticaria, eczema, allergic rhinitis.
- Chronic inflammatory conditions especially autoimmune disorders and chronic infections.

- Acute infections, possibly retroviral infections.
- Hypertension.
- Atherosclerosis (prophylaxis also).
- Cataract and diabetic complications.
- Restless foetus and toxaemia of pregnancy.

Dosage

2 to 6 g/day of the dried root or 4 to 12mL/day of 1:2 fluid extract.

REFERENCES

1   Bensky, D and Gamble, A: *Chinese Herbal Medicine Materia Medica*, Eastland Press, Seattle (1986).
2   Chang, H M et al: *Advances in Chinese Medicinal Materials Research*, World Scientific, Singapore (1985).
3   Tang, W and Eisenbrand, G: *Chinese Drugs of Plant Origin*, Springer Verlag, Berlin (1992).
4   Amellal, M et al: *Planta Medica* **51**, 16 (1985).
5   Li, Z et al: *Chin J Integ Trad West Med* **9**, 698 (1989) in *Abst Chin Med* **3**, 395 (1989).
6   Chang, H M and But, P P: *Pharmacology and Applications of Chinese Materia Medica*, Vol 2, World Scientific, Singapore (1987).
7   Kimura, Y et al: *Planta Medica* **51**, 132 (1985).
8   Kimura, Y et al: *Biochim Biophys Acta* **922**, 278 (1987).
9   Kimura, Y et al: *Chem Pharm Bull (Tokyo)* **34**, 2279 (1986).
10 Butenko, I G et al: *Agents and Actions* **39**, 49 (1993).
11 Cheng, C P et al: *Planta Medica* **61**, 150 (1995).
12 Umeda, M et al: *J Ethnopharmacol* **23**, 91 (1988).
13 Kubo, M et al: *Chem Pharm Bull (Tokyo)* **33**, 2411 (1985).
14 Kimura, Y et al: *Chem Pharm Bull (Tokyo)* **29**, 2610 (1981).
15 Hara, H et al: *Eur J Pharmacol* **221**, 193 (1992).
16 Nakayama, S et al: *Nippon Yakurigaku Zasshi* **101**, 327 (1993).
17 Hamada, H et al: *Arch Biochem Biophys* **306**, 261 (1993).
18 Li, B Q et al: *Cell Molec Biol Res* **39**, 119 (1993).
19 Bae, K H et al: *Planta Medica* **60**, 280 (1994).
20 Motoo, Y and Sawabu, N: *Cancer Letters* **86**, 91 (1994).
21 Huang, H C et al: *Eur J Pharmacol* **268,** 73 (1994).
22 Huang, H C et al: *Eur J Pharmacol* **251,** 91 (1994).
23 Seki, T and Morohashi, M: *Skin Pharmacol* **6**, 56 (1993).
24 Chen, S et al: *Arch Biochem Biophys* **302**, 72 (1993).
25 Natarajan, R et al: *Hypertension* **23**, 142 (1994).
26 Bell-Quilley C P et al: *J Pharmacol Exp Therapeut* **267**, 676 (1993).
27 Wu, S H et al: *Kidney Internat* **43**, 1280 (1993).
28 Bone, K: *Baical Skullcap* MediHerb Professional Newsletter, July (1993) MediHerb Pty Ltd, Warwick.
29 Abe, K et al: *Chem Bull Pharm (Tokyo)* **38**, 209 (1990).
30 Nagai, H et al: *Jap J Pharmacol* **25**, 763 (1975).
31 Lin, W S et al: *Shanghai J Trad Chin Med* **1**, 22 (1987) in *Abst Chin Med* **2**, 57 (1988).

Stephania tetrandra

Mandarin	Han Fang Ji
Family	Menispermaceae
Part Used	Root

Properties

Bitter, acrid and cold. Stephania is diuretic, antirheumatic and analgesic and is used for rheumatism, rheumatoid arthritis, oedema and dysuria.[1]

Active Constituents

The root contains many isoquinoline alkaloids, the major one being a bis-benzylisoquinoline alkaloid known as tetrandrine (0.6–0.9%).[2] The root also contains flavonoids.

Tetrandrine

Pharmacology of Tetrandrine and Related Alkaloids

→ *Calcium Channel Antagonist*

- Recent studies have indicated tetrandrine is a blocker of the voltage-activated, L-type calcium channel in cardiac, anterior pituitary and neuroblastoma cells and in rat neurohypophyseal nerve terminals. Its binding site is located at the benzothiazepine receptor on the alpha 1-subunit of the channel. It also blocks the voltage-dependent T-type calcium channel. This blocking explains tetrandrine's application to cardiovascular diseases. Tetrandrine has also demonstrated the unusual ability to block the calcium-activated potassium channels of neurohypophyseal nerve terminals.[3]

- Tetrandrine and isotetrandrine relaxed the contractile response caused by depolarizing solution or noradrenaline. Both alkaloids did not affect caffeine-induced contraction. The refilling of intracellular calcium stores sensitive to noradrenaline or caffeine was inhibited by both alkaloids.[4]

- Tetrandine may inhibit monocyte migration into arterial subendothelial space through antagonism to calcium and thereby suppress atherogenesis.[5]

- The calcium channel antagonism of tetrandrine probably explains the following observations:

CARDIOVASCULAR ACTIVITY

- Tetrandrine counters the tonic effect of calcium on the myocardium.[6]

- Tetrandrine counters cardiac arrhythmias induced by toxic agents and is analogous to the drug verapamil.[6]

- Tetrandrine dilates coronary vessels.[1]

- Tetrandrine has significant hypotensive action and is under study as a new hypotensive drug. Other alkaloids in the root may even be more potent.[1]

SMOOTH MUSCLE

- Tetrandrine relaxed the chemically induced tension in rat tail artery *in vitro.*[7]

STRIATED MUSCLE

- All the alkaloids of the root are potent striated muscle relaxants.[1]

➡ *Anti-inflammatory, Antiallergic Effects*

IN VITRO

- Tetrandrine is a potent inhibitor of cellular involvement in inflammation and allergic reaction.[8]

- Tetrandrine suppresses phagocytosis, especially monocytes. It also demonstrated potent antioxidant properties. Suppression of cellular immunity may be caused by Ca antagonism.[9,10]

- Tetrandrine inhibited both interleukin-1 production and activity.[11]

- Tetrandrine is more potent than berbamine in terms of inhibitory effects on production of interleukin-1 and tumour necrosis factors by macrophages and lymphocytes.[12]

- Tetrandrine inhibited the production of leukotriene B_4 and thromboxane B_2. The effects were similar to that of a calmodulin antagonist.[13]

- Tetrandrine inhibits mast cell degranulation.[14]

- Tetrandrine inhibited antibody synthesis, natural killer cells and mitogen-induced lymphoproliferation.[15]

- Several bisbenzylisoquinoline alkaloids including tetrandrine and isotetrandrine suppressed nitric oxide production by macrophages. (Nitric oxide is a mediator in inflammation).[16]

IN VIVO

- Tetrandrine suppressed the chronic inflammation in adjuvant-induced arthritis in rats but was not active in an acute inflammation test. Timing of the administration was important in reducing the signs of arthritis. Oral doses of tetrandrine were more potent than aspirin, without the gastric irritation.[17]

- Tetrandrine demonstrated an anti-inflammatory action in carrageenin-induced pleurisy in rats. Intra-gastric administration of tetrandrine reduced inflammatory parameters such as phospholipase A_2 activity.[18]

- Tetrandrine was investigated for its effects on asthma and allergic inflammation in guinea pigs. Significant inhibition of microvascular leakage by tetrandrine was observed with all four allergic mediators.[19]

- Tetrandrine was found to be a more potent suppressant of platelet-activating-factor-induced mononuclear cell infiltration, but less potent in carrageenin-induced polymorphonuclear leukocyte infiltration.[20]

- Tetrandrine inhibited monokine release from both silica- and lipopolysaccharide-stimulated alveolar macrophages. Tetrandrine also inhibited interleukin-1-mediated thymocyte proliferation *in vitro*. These results provide a correlation between the antifibrotic effect of tetrandrine and inhibition of macrophage activation.[21]

- Tetrandrine and berbamine reduced the incidence of relapsing experimental allergic encephalitis in rats by 41 and 65% respectively.[22]

- Tetrandrine was investigated as a pulpotomy medicament. Lymphocyte infiltration was reduced in teeth treated with tetrandrine in comparison to treatment with orthodox drugs and controls. Both acute and chronic inflammation was reduced.[23]

- Injection of tetrandrine demonstrated an inhibitory effect on experimental uveitis in rabbits. Tetrandrine did not produce a withdrawal rebound.[24]

➡ *Antifibrotic and Pulmonary Effects*

- Tetrandrine effectively blocks the ability of quartz to stimulate oxidant release from pulmonary phagocytes, thus reducing damage to lung cells in pulmonary fibrosis.[25]

- Tetrandrine inhibited the development of experimental silicosis in rats and the synthesis of collagen in rat lung. Further studies suggest that both tetrandrine and an antisilicotic compound inhibit the gene expression of collagen during silicosis.[26]

- A recent study suggests the mechanism governing the antifibrotic action of tetrandrine may be mediated in part by direct inhibition of fibroblast proliferation normally associated with the development and progression of silicosis.[27]

- The effect of tetrandrine was studied on rabbits with smoke inhalation injury. Tetrandrine decreased the pulmonary and tracheal vascular permeability, lung oedema and improved respiratory function.[28]

- The lipid content of lung tissues of rats with experimental silicosis was lower than that of untreated animals.[29]

- Tetrandrine showed strong binding to both lipid vesicles and alveolar macrophages.[30]

➡ *Immunologic Function*

- Delayed administration of tetrandrine to young rats reduced the cumulative incidence of diabetes from 73 to 42%. Combination of tetrandrine with an immunosuppressive drug reduced the incidence to only 4%. This combination may represent an effective treatment for patients with recent or imminent insulin dependent diabetes mellitus.[31] An earlier study demonstrated that if administration of tetrandrine (20 mg/kg/day) was delayed until 70 days of age, the incidence of diabetes was reduced from 63 to 29%.[32]

- Tetrandrine injected intraperitoneally protected rats from chemically-induced diabetes. Tetrandrine prevented damage to pancreatic beta cells.[33]

- Tetrandrine showed potent inhibition of respiratory burst activity *in vitro*. The mechanism by which bisbenzylisoquinoline alkaloids inhibit activation of phagocytes is likely to involve cellular microtubules and microfilaments.[34]

- Plaque-forming cell response in mice to antigens was suppressed by low dose tetrandrine. Tetrandrine exerts selective inhibition of T-cell-dependent immune reactions.[35]

- Although tetrandrine is not cytotoxic to phagocytic cells, it is a potent inhibitor *in vitro* of stimulant-induced activation of phagocytic cells.[36]

- Tetrandrine and berbamine are equipotent in terms of antibody responses and suppression of delayed-type hypersensitivity (DTH) responses to antigens. Although the alkaloids did not affect antibody responses in experimental brucellosis in mice, they caused equipotent suppression of DTH. Berbamine enhanced spleen colony counts.[37]

➜ Other Effects

- Oral administration of tetrandrine reduced mortality in spontaneously hypertensive rats by 22%. Tetrandrine decreased the severity of ventricular hypertrophy.[38]
- Tetrandrine has a mild analgesic effect and kills cancer cells *in vitro* and *in vivo*.[1]
- Tetrandrine caused the death of malignant lymphoid and myeloid cells but not Epstein-Barr virus-transformed lymphoblastoid cells *in vitro*.[39]
- Isotetrandrine potently inhibited the experimentally-induced activation of polymorphonuclear leucocytes *in vitro*.[40]

Toxicity

- Tetrandrine has a very low oral toxicity e.g. 2.2 g/kg in rats.[1] Other alkaloids in the root are considerably more toxic, but the oral toxicity of the root is still very low at 240 g/kg in mice.

Clinical Studies

➜ Cardiovascular Conditions

- Tetrandrine at 100 mg three times daily orally, significantly reduced blood pressure within 1 week (equivalent to 10 to 20g herb/day). Blood pressure has also been lowered using the root in combination with other herbs.[1]
- Good results were obtained in angina for injection of tetrandrine.[1]
- An open clinical trial investigated the electrophysiologic effect of intravenous tetrandrine on 20 patients. The effective rate on supraventricular tachycardia (SVT) was 86%, curative effect on atrioventricular nodal re-entrant tachycardia was 100% and on atrioventricular re-entrant tachycardia, 71%. Tetrandrine prevented induction of SVT in 4 cases, and 4 cases of sustained SVT were no longer sustained.[41]
- Tetrandrine was given to nine patients with pulmonary hypertension secondary to chronic obstructive pulmonary disease. Sixty minutes after administration, total pulmonary vascular resistance and pulmonary artery mean pressure were reduced by 23% and 15% respectively. There was no change in the cardiac output.[42]

- Diastolic and systolic functions of 34 hypertensive patients were studied. Left ventricular (LV) hypertrophy is one of the important factors in impairing LV diastolic function in essential hypertension. Intravenous administration of verapamil and tetrandrine improved LV diastolic function without any apparent adverse influence on systolic function.[43]

- An open clinical trial was conducted on 38 patients, most with essential hypertension. Patients were treated with oral tetrandrine for 1 month with a total effective rate of 92%, the "marked improvement" rate being 63%. No postural hypotension or other serious side effects were observed.[44]

➜ *Silicosis*

- Tetrandrine has been shown to retard and even sometimes reverse the inflammatory and fibrotic lesions of pulmonary silicosis.[15]

➜ *Other Conditions*

- Oral tetrandrine at 40mg three times daily for 10 days was effective in both acute and chronic amoebic dysentery.[1]

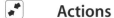 ## Actions

Anti-inflammatory, muscle relaxant, hypotensive, antiarrhythmic, antiallergic, immunodepressant, diuretic, antifibrotic.

Medicinal Uses of Stephania

- High blood pressure, angina, arrythmias.
- Rheumatoid arthritis, pulmonary silicosis.
- Autoimmune diseases, chronic inflammation, allergies.
- Acute and chronic amoebic dysentery.
- Oedema especially in the lower body.
- Use cautiously as is a powerful herb, especially at higher doses.

Dosage

2 to 10 g/day of the dried root, or 4 to 12 mL/day of the 1:2 fluid extract, caution with higher doses.

REFERENCES

1 Chang, H M and But P P: *Phamacology and Applications of Chinese Materia Medica*, Vol 1, World Scientific, Singapore (1986).

2 Yang, Y F et al: *Bull Chin Materia Medica* **13**, 740 (1988) in *Abst Chin Med* **3**, 15 (1989).

3 Wang, G and Lemos J R: *Life Sci* **56**, 295 (1995).

4   Anselmi, E et al: *Pharmazie* **49**, 440 (1994).

5   Zhou, X: *Chung-Hua I Hsueh Tsa Chih* **72**, 424, 447 (1992).

6   Fang, D C et al: *Chin Med J* **99**, 638 (1986).

7   Liu, Q Y et al: *J Pharmacol Exp Therapeut* **273**, 32 (1995).

8   Seow, W K et al: *Immunol Lett* **13**, 83 (1986).

9   Seow, W K et al: *Int Arch Allergy Appl Immunol* **85**, 404 (1988).

10 Seow, W K et al: *Clin Exp Immunol* **75**, 47 (1989).

11 Chang, M L et al: *J Microbiol Immunol* **26**, 15 (1993).

12 Seow, W K et al: *Life Sci* **50**, PL53 (1992).

13 Du, Z Y and Huang, Y H: *Chung-Kuo Yao Li Hseuh Pao* **14**, 325 (1993).

14 Li, W et al: *Acta Pharmacol Sin* **8**, 450 (1987) in *Abst Chin Med* **2**, 153 (1988).

15 Seow, W K et al: *Int Arch Allergy Appl Immunol* **85**, 410 (1988).

16 Kondo, Y et al: *Biochem Pharmacol* **46**, 1887 (1993).

17 Whitehouse, M W et al: *Agents & Actions* **42**, 123 (1994).

18 He, H M et al: *Chung-Kuo Yao Li Hseuh Pao* **15**, 477 (1994).

19 Wong, C W et al: *Int J Immunopharmacol* **15**, 185 (1993).

20 Wong, C W et al: *Agents & Actions* **36**, 112 (1992).

21 Kang, J H et al: *Exp Lung Res* **18**, 715 (1992).

22 Wong, C W et al: *Int Arch Allergy Immunol* **97**, 31 (1992).

23 Seow, W K and Thong, Y H: *Pediatric Dentistry* **15**, 260 (1993).

24 Xiao, J et al: *J Ocular Pharmacol* **9**, 151 (1993).

25 Castranova, V: *Envir Health Perspectives* **102**, 65 (1994).

26 Liu, B C et al: *Biomed Envir Sci* **7**, 199 (1994).

27 Reist, R H et al: *Toxicol Appl Pharmacol* **122**, 70 (1993).

28 Zhang, M: *Chung-Hua Cheng Hsing Shao Shang Wai Ko Tsa Chih* **9**, 121, 160 (1993).

29 San, S et al: *Biomed Environ Sci* **5**, 362 (1992).

30 Ma, J K et al: *Exp Lung Res* **17**, 1061 (1991).

31 Lieberman, I et al: *Life Sci* **53**, PL 453 (1993).

32 Lieberman, I et al: *Diabetes* **41**, 616 (1992).

33 Sun, G R et al: *Sheng Li Hseuh Pao* **46**, 161 (1994).

34 Ma, J Y et al: *Exp Lung Res* **18**, 829 (1992).

35 Kondo, Y et al: *Int J Immunopharmacol* **14**, 1181 (1992).

36 Castranova, V et al: *J Leukocyte Biol* **50**, 412 (1991).

37 Wong, C W et al: *Int J Immunopharm* **13**, 579 (1991).

38 Chen, H et al: *Int J Cardiol* **41**, 103 (1993).

39 Teh, B S et al: *Int J Immunopharmacol* **13**, 1117 (1991).

40 Kinoshita, K et al: *Planta Medica* **58**, 137 (1992).

41 Li W H: *Chung-Hua Hsin Hsueh Kuan Ping Tsa Chih* **21**, 225, 254 (1993).

42 Kang, J: *Chung-Hua Chieh Ho Ho Hu Hsi Tsa Chih* **16**, 93, 124 (1993).

43 Zeng, B and Dai, G Z: *Chung-Hua Nei Ko Tsa Chih* **30**, 134, 187 (1991).

44 Anonymous: *Chin Med J* **92**, 193 (1979).

Zizyphus jujuba var spinosa

Also known as *Zizyphus spinosa*.

Mandarin	Suan Zao Ren
English	Sour Chinese Date Seed
Family	Rhamnaceae
Part Used	Seed

Properties

Sweet and mild. Zizyphus is sedative and antihydrotic and is used for insomnia due to nervous exhaustion and anxiety, palpitations and excessive sweating.

Active Constituents

Saponins such as jujubosides A and B,[1] fixed oil and volatile oil.

Jujuboside A

Pharmacology

→ *Sedative and Hypnotic Effects*

- Sedative effects have been demonstrated on many animals by various tests.[2]
- Zizyphus has synergistic effects with many sedatives and hypnotics.[2]
- The active components are thought to be the jujubosides.

→ *Other Effects*

- The herb is also anticonvulsant, hypotensive and prolongs survival after burns. It has very low toxicity and also improved hypoxia tolerance in rats.[2]

Clinical Studies

- Suanzaorentang is a formula containing mainly Zizyphus. It has been studied in double-blind trials. One study of patients with anxiety found that it significantly improved mood, decreased sympathetic nervous system symptoms and improved performance.[3] Another study of insomnia showed a significant improvement in sleep quality and well-being without side effects.[4]

Actions

Sedative, hypnotic, hypotensive.

Medicinal Uses

- Anxiety, insomnia, nervous exhaustion, irritability, palpitations.
- Hypertension and excessive sweating in the anxious patient, night sweats.

Dosage

2 to 8 g/day of the dried seed or 4 to 16 mL/day of the 1:2 fluid extract.

REFERENCES

1   Tang, W and Eisenbrand, G: *Chinese Drugs of Plant Origin*, Springer Verlag, Berlin (1992).
2   Chang, H M and But, P P: *Pharmacology and Applications of Chinese Materia Medica* Vol 2, World Scientific, Singapore (1987).
3   Chen, H C et al: *Int J Chin Pharmacol Therapeut Toxicol* **24**, 646 (1986).
4   Chen, H C and Hsieh, M T: *Clin Therapeut* **7**, 335 (1985).

Ayurvedic Herbs

Adhatoda vasica

Also known as *Justicia adhatoda*.

Sanskrit	Amalaka
English	Malabar Nut Tree
Family	Acanthaceae
Part Used	Leaves

A small evergreen bush which grows commonly in open plains, especially in the lower Himalayas.

Active Constituents

Essential oil (0.08%) and about 1% alkaloids including vasicine, vasicinone and vasicinol. Vasicine, which comprises around 75 to 90% of the total alkaloids is considered to be the major active constituent.[1]

Vasicine   Vasicinone

Pharmacology

→ *Bronchial Effects*

- Early work found a mild bronchodilating effect from an alkaloid similar in action to atropine (vagus depression).

- Some recent work has demonstrated contrary effects: that vasicine and vasicinone are mild potentiators of acetylcholine and therefore cause bronchoconstriction.[2]

- Other work has found vasicine to be a bronchodilator and respiratory stimulant.[3]
- The drug bromhexine (Bisolvon) was developed from vasicine and is used as an aid to expectoration through reducing the viscosity of secretions.[3,4]
- Additional respiratory studies on Adhatoda found:[5]
  - Antiasthmatic activity.
  - Protection against histamine-induced bronchospasm.
  - Confirmation of the respiratory stimulant effect of vasicine.
  - Vasicine increases ciliary movement (expectorant effect).
  - The whole alkaloid complex of the herb is likely to be bronchodilatory, especially if the bronchi are in a contracted state.
- The alkaloids from Adhatoda (10 mg/mL aerosol) showed pronounced protection against allergen-induced bronchial obstruction in guinea pigs.[6]

➜ Uterine Activity

- A potent activity for vasicine has been demonstrated on the pregnant or non-pregnant uterus. It is similar to oxytocin in that its effect is more pronounced in late pregnancy and immediately after birth. Vasicine potentiates the effect of oxytocin and probably acts through the release of endogenous prostaglandins.[7]
- Aqueous-ethanol extract of Adhatoda showed 100% abortifacient activity in a recent study in rats orally dosed with 175 mg/kg.[8]
- Vasicine is oxidised by the liver to vasicinone. This means that oral doses have a low oxytocic activity but that the bronchial activities are not greatly affected.[5]

Clinical Studies

- Clinical studies showed an expectorant action, especially in acute bronchitis with a loosening of thick phlegm. Benefits in asthma are as much due to expectorant and antiallergic effects as to bronchodilation.
- Significant improvement in the inflammation and bleeding of gums was noted in 25 patients after the application of *Adhatoda vasica* extract.[9]

Actions

Expectorant, bronchodilator, antiasthmatic, oxytocic.

Medicinal Uses

- Respiratory diseases such as asthma and acute and chronic bronchitis.
- Post-partum haemorrage and to assist uterine involution.

- Locally for gum disease (proven in clinical trial).[9]
- Contraindicated in pregnancy except at birth.

Dosage

0.5 to 1.5 g/day of the dried herb or 1 to 3 mL/day of the 1:2 extract. May need higher doses for the oxytocic effect and to increase the bioavailability of vasicine using *Piper longum*. Also can be used as douche for the oxytocic effect. Unlikely that abortifacient doses can be achieved by oral use of the herb, but it is best to be cautious.

REFERENCES

1   Pundarikakshudu, K and Bharsar, G C: *Int J Crude Drug Res* **26**, 88 (1988)

2   Lahiri, P K et al: *Indian J Exp Biol* **2**, 220 (1964)

3   Gupta O P et al: *Indian J Med Res* **66**, 680 (1977)

4   Bruce, R A and Kumar, V: *Brit J Clin Pract* **22**, 289 (1968)

5   Atal, C K: *Chemistry and Pharmacology of Vasicine A New Oxytocic and Abortifacient,* Regional Research, Jammu-Tawi (1980)

6   Dorsch, W: *Int Arch Allergy Appl Immunol* **94**, 262 (1991)

7   Gupta, O P et al: *Indian J Med Res* **66**, 865 (1977)

8   Nath, D et al: *J Ethnopharmacol* **36**, 147 (1992)

9   Doshi, J J et al: *Int J Crude Drug Res* **21**, 173 (1983)

Albizzia lebbeck

Sanskrit	Pit Shirish Shirisha
Family	Leguminosae — Mimosa subgroup
Part Used	Stem bark

Active Constituents

Not well-defined. Saponins and cardiac glycosides, tannins, flavonoids. Does not contain alkaloids.

Pharmacology

- Has antifungal and antibacterial activity.
- Spasmolytic on intestinal smooth muscle.[1]
- Positively inotropic in isolated heart preparations.[1]
- Early studies showed partial protection against histamine and acetylcholine-induced bronchoconstriction.[1]
- Albizzia also protected against the effects of antigen challenge.[1]
- In a series of studies[1,2] effects on allergy mechanisms were further investigated. The following results were observed for oral doses of 25 mg/kg/day for 7–12 days:
  - A stabilizing effect on mast cells when compared to disodium cromoglycate (Intal) and steroids (prednisolone). Degranulation was inhibited by 62%.
  - Early processes of sensitisation were also inhibited.
  - Levels of allergy-inducing antibodies were depressed.
  - Active constituents were heat-stable and water-soluble.
  - The herb also significantly decreased serum cholesterol.
  - T-lymphocyte activity and possibly B-lymphocyte activity were depressed.
- Albizzia (150 mg/kg, oral) had a 75% protective effect against anaphylactic shock in guinea pigs, whereas Intal had no effect.[2]
- In a later study[3] the effect of quercetin, a crude extract of Albizzia seeds and a pure saponin fraction of Albizzia were studied on mast cells. All substances had

a membrane stabilizing effect on mast cells from the mesentery and peritoneal fluid of rats subjected to anaphylaxis.

Clinical Studies

- In an uncontrolled study in 60 patients with asthma it was found that clinical response depended on the duration of the disease. Response was excellent for asthma of recent onset (less than two years). Results were less predictable in older cases.[1]

- Local application in cases of weeping eczema produced marked improvement.[1]

- Preliminary trials for allergic rhinitis showed promising results.[1]

Actions

Antiallergic, hypocholesterolaemic, antimicrobial, possibly cardiotonic.

Medicinal Uses

- Traditionally used for respiratory diseases including asthma and skin diseases such as eczema.

- Atopic allergy — allergic rhinitis, asthma, eczema (including topically), urticaria.

- May be useful for high blood cholesterol.

Dosage

3 to 6 mL/day of the 1:2 extract. Higher doses by decoction.

REFERENCES

1   Tripathi, R M et al: *J Ethnopharmacol* **1**, 385 (1979)
2   Tripathi, R M et al: *J Ethnopharmacol* **1**, 397 (1979)
3   Johri, R K et al: *Indian J Physiol Pharmacol* **29**, 43 (1985)

Andrographis paniculata

Sanskrit	Kirata
Bengali	Kalmegh
English	Chiretta, King of Bitters
Family	Acanthaceae
Part Used	Herb

An annual plant common throughout the plains of India. Also cultivated in gardens. Andrographis is also used in traditional Chinese Medicine and was originally imported into China.

Active Constituents

Bitter diterpenoid lactones (andrographolides), diterpene glucosides, diterpene dimers,[1] flavonoids including TFAP.[2]

Andrographolide

⁙ Pharmacology

➔ *Immunologic Function and Infestation*

- Although Andrographis is widely used in infections and infestations, the weight of evidence is that its value here is mainly as an immune-enhancing treatment. Early reports attributed an antibacterial activity to the plant which has not recently been confirmed. The andrographolides are devoid of antibacterial activity.[3]

- Blood samples collected from 10 healthy volunteers who received oral doses of Andrographis showed no evidence of bactericidal activity. Similar results were found in animal studies.[4]

- Subcutaneous administration of a water decoction of Andrographis leaves to infected animals reduced nematode larvae in the blood by 85%.[5]

- Fluid extract of Andrographis root demonstrated strong *in vitro* anthelmintic activity against human *Ascaris lumbricoides*.[6]

- An immunostimulant action, especially on phagocytosis has been demonstrated.[3]

- Andrographis fluid extract and isolated andrographolide stimulated both antigen-specific and non-specific immune responses in mice. The fluid extract produced stronger immunostimulation.[7]

- Dehydroandrographolide succinic acid monoester (DASM), a drug derived from andrographolide, has been found to inhibit HIV *in vitro*. This effect was observed on several HIV strains and DASM was non-toxic to other cells in the concentration range. However, dehydroandrographolide was devoid of anti-HIV activity.[8]

- Prolonged survival in animals after snakebite was observed after pretreatment with extracts of Andrographis.[9]

➔ *Hepatoprotective and Choleretic Activities*

- Oral administration of Andrographis extract and andrographolide to rats demonstrated a protective action against CCl4-induced hepatic toxicity. The leaf extract showed stronger activity than andrographolide.[10]

- In Ayurveda, Andrographis is primarily a liver herb and choleretic and hepatoprotective effects have been demonstrated.[11,12]

- Andrographolide produced a dose-dependent choleretic effect (increased bile flow, bile salt and bile acids) in animals. The effect was stronger than silymarin.[12]

- Andrographolide showed protective activity against chemically-induced toxicity on rat hepatocytes *in vitro*. The hepatoprotective effect was greater than silymarin.[13]

- Three diterpene constituents of Andrographis showed protective effects on hepatotoxicity induced in mice by various chemicals. The protective effect of andrographiside and neoandrographolide was as strong as silymarin, and could be due to the glucoside groups acting as strong antioxidants.[14]

- Andrographolide exhibited hepatoprotective activity after oral or ip administration to rats with chemically-induced acute hepatitis. Treatment with the herb led to complete nomalization of 5 biochemical parameters and improved the histopathological changes in the liver.[15]

➡ *Cardiovascular Activity*

- Andrographis was found to alleviate myocardial ischaemic reperfusion injury.[16]

- A study on rabbits found Andrographis to alleviate atherosclerotic artery stenosis induced by both de-endothelialization and a high cholesterol diet.[17] In addition, it lowered the restenosis rate after experimental angioplasty.[17]

- TFAP has anti-inflammatory and antiplatelet effects which prevent the development of myocardial infarction.[2] An earlier study using an aqueous extract iv suggested that Andrographis may limit the expansion of the ischaemic focus, exert a marked protective effect on reversible ischaemic myocardium and demonstrate a weak fibrinolytic action.[18]

➡ *Antifertility Activity*

- Oral administration of Andrographis leaf powder (20 mg/day for 60 days) to male rats produced an antifertility effect possibly due to an antispermatogenic and/or antiandrogenic mechanism.[19]

- A controlled experiment in female mice fed with 2g/kg/day found Andrographis prevented pregnancy in 100% of those treated.[20]

➡ *Other Effects*

- Several studies have shown antipyretic and anti-inflammatory effects for the andrographolides.[3]

- Alcoholic extract of Andrographis showed potent cell differentiation-inducing activity on mouse leukemia cells.[1]

- Studies have implied that the andrographolides promote ACTH and consequently enhance adrenocortical function.[3]

- The following studies demonstrate potentially conflicting activities:

  – Aqueous extract of Andrographis (10 mg/kg) was found to prevent glucose-induced hyperglycaemia in rabbits. It failed to prevent hyperglycaemia induced by adrenalin, suggesting that the herb prevents glucose absorption from the gut.[21]

  – Oral administration of Andrographis extract and andrographolide produced a dose- and time-dependent activation of brush-border membrane-bound hydrolases in rats. This suggests Andrographis accelerates intestinal digestion and absorption of carbohydrate (as opposed to simple glucose by activation of these intestinal disaccharidases).[22]

Clinical Studies

• Enteric infections: many Chinese studies of acute bacillary dysentery and enteritis have shown a marked benefit.[3]

• Clinical studies in bacterial and viral respiratory infections demonstrated good effects, implying an immunostimulant action.[3]

• A randomized double blind study on 152 patients with pharyngotonsillitis found 6g/day of Andrographis for a week to be as effective as paracetamol in providing relief of fever and sore throat. Lower doses of Andrographis were not as effective.[23]

• Leptospirosis, snake bite, acute pyelonephritis, tuberculosis and leprosy have also responded to treatment with Andrographis.[3]

• A study on patients with cardiac and cerebral vascular disease found that Andrographis inhibited platelet aggregation induced by ADP. Serotonin released from platelets was decreased, but plasma serotonin levels remained unchanged.[24]

Actions

Bitter tonic, choleretic, immunostimulant, hepatoprotective, antipyretic, anti-inflammatory, abortifacient, possibly adaptogen.

Adverse Effects

High doses may cause gastric discomfort, anorexia and emesis, but generally there are few side effects and it is non-toxic.

Medicinal Uses

• Acute and chronic infections, weakened immunity, worm infestation. Traditionally was considered to be superior to quinine in malaria.

• Toxic liver damage, liver infections, poor liver function.

- May have value in cardiovascular disease.
- Contraindicated in pregnancy.

 ## Dosage

1.5 to 6 g/day of dried herb, or 3 to 12 mL/day of 1:2 fluid extract.

REFERENCES

1   Matsuda, T et al: *Chem and Pharm Bull (Tokyo)* **42**, 1216 (1994)

2   Zhao, H Y and Fang W Y: *Chinese Med J* **104**, 770 (1991)

3   Chang H M and But P P: *Pharmacology and Applications of Chinese Materia Medica*, Vol 2, World Scientific, Singapore (1987)

4   Leelarasamee, A et al: *J Med Assoc Thailand* **73**, 299 (1990)

5   Dutta, A and Sukul, N C: *J Helminthology* **56**, 81 (1982)

6   Raj, R K: *Ind J Physiol Pharmacol* **19**, (1975)

7   Puri, A et al: *J Natural Products* **56**, 995 (1993)

8   Chang, R S et al: *Proc Soc Exp Biol Med* **197**, 59 (1991)

9   Martz, W: *Toxicon* **30**, 1131 (1992)

10 Choudhury, B R and Poddar, M K: *Meth Find Exp Clin Pharm* **6**, 481 (1984)

11 Tripathi, G S and Tripathi Y B: *Phytotherapy Res* **5**, 176 (1991)

12 Shukla, B et al: *Planta Medica* **58**, 146 (1992)

13 Visen, P K et al: *J Ethnopharmacology* **40**, 131 (1993)

14 Kapril, A et al: *Biochemical Pharmacology* **46**, 182 (1993)

15 Handa, S S and Sharma, A: *Ind J Med Res* **92**, 284 (1990)

16 Guo, Z L et al: *J Tongji Med University* **14**, 49 (1994)

17 Wang, D W and Zhao H Y: *Chinese Med J* **107**, 464 (1994)

18 Zhao, H Y and Fang W Y: *J Tongji Med University* **10**, 212 (1990)

19 Akbarsha, M A et al: *Ind J Exp Biol* **28**, 421 (1990)

20 Zoha, M S et al: *Banglasdesh Med Res Council Bull* **15**, 34 (1989)

21 Borhanuddin, M et al: *Bangadesh Med Res Council Bull* **20**, 24 (1994)

22 Choudhury, B R and Poddar, M K: *Meth Find Exp Clin Pharm* **7**, 617 (1985)

23 Thamlikitkul, V et al: *J Med Assoc Thailand* **74**, 437 (1991)

24 Zhang Y Z et al: *Chung-Kuo Chung Hsi I Chieh Ho Tsa Chin* **14**, 5, 28, 34 (1994)

Bacopa monniera

Also known as *Herpestis monniera*.

Sanskrit	Brahmi
Family	Scrophulariaceae
Parts Used	Herb or whole plant

An annual succulent creeping plant found throughout India in wet, damp and marshy areas. Often confused with Gotu Kola (*Centella asiatica*) which is also known as Brahmi. Bacopa is the foremost nerve tonic of Ayurveda traditionally used for epilepsy, insanity, and to improve memory and mental capacities. It is also native to Australia.

Active Constituents

Like Centella, these are mainly saponins — the major ones being the steroidal saponins Bacoside A and B.[1]

Pharmacology

- In an early study the saponin fraction was shown to have cardiotonic, vasoconstricting and sedative activities.[2]

- Another study compared Bacopa and chlorpromazine on the learning process in rats.[3] Both improved performance in the learning phase, but did not improve performance in animals with well-established habits. Chlorpromazine depressed motor efficiency, but no such deleterious effects were observed for Bacopa — in fact it improved motor efficiency compared to controls.

- More recent studies have also looked at the effect of Bacopa on learning ability in rats.[4] In one study 200 mg/kg was given orally for 3 days prior to commencement, then a support dose of 200 mg/kg was given every third day. Results were as follows:

  - In a brightness-discrimination reaction, Brahmi improved acquisition, retention, and delayed extinction of the newly acquired behaviour.

  - In active conditioned flight reaction, the rats with Bacopa took 6 days to learn the response whereas control animals took 10.

– In continuous avoidance response, the Bacopa-treated animals learnt quicker and were fully adapted after 20 days whereas controls had not adapted.

- A formula known as Brahmi Rasayan consisting of 10 parts Bacopa, 2 parts Cloves, 1 part Cardamon, 1 part *Piper longum*, and 40 parts sucrose was studied in mice and rats.[5] High doses showed the following effects:

  – Sedative with no effect on motor co-ordination

  – Analgesic

  – Anticonvulsant

- In a recent study, oral doses (1–10 g/kg) of Brahmi Rasayan were found to suppress experimentally induced inflammation.[6] The herbal formula did not produce gastric irritation.

Clinical Studies

- An open clinical study on 13 patients with epilepsy using the defatted, alcoholic extract of Bacopa demonstrated improvements in the frequency of fitting over 2 to 5 months. The onset of epileptic fits was completely checked in 5 cases.[7]

Actions

Nervine tonic, mild sedative, mild anticonvulsant, anti-inflammatory.

Medicinal Uses

- As a brain tonic for improving memory, concentration and learning.
- Nervous deficit due to injury and stroke.
- Nervous breakdown, nervous exhaustion.
- May be of value in epilepsy and insanity.

Dosage

2 to 6 g/day of the dried herb or 4 to 12 mL/day of the 1:2 extract.

REFERENCES

1 Chatterji, N et al: *Indian J Chem* **3**, 24 (1965)

2 Malhotra, C L and Das, P K: *Indian J Med Res* **47**, 294 (1959)

3 Prakash, J C and Sirsi, M: *J Sci Industr Res* **21C**, 93 (1962)

4 Singh, H K and Dhawan, B N: *J Ethnopharmacol* **5**, 205 (1982)

5 Shukia, B et al: *J Ethnopharmacol* **21**, 65 (1987)

6 Jain, P et al: *Indian J Exp Biol* **32**, 633 (1994)

7 Mukherjee, G D and Dey, C D: *J Exp Med Sc* **11**, 82 (1968)

Coleus forskohlii

Sanskrit	Makandi
Family	Lamiaceae
Part Used	Root

A small member of the Lamiaceae (Labiatae) which grows as a perennial on the Indian plains and lower Himalayas. It is also grown as an ornamental and the root is used as a spice.

Active Constituents

Essential oil and diterpenes, especially the labdane diterpene forskolin (0.2 to 0.3%), which is also known as coleonol.

Forskolin

Pharmacology of Forskolin

- Activation of adenylate cyclase through direct stimulation of the catalytic subunit[1] (see below). This characteristic property of forskolin has led to its extensive use as a biochemical tool.

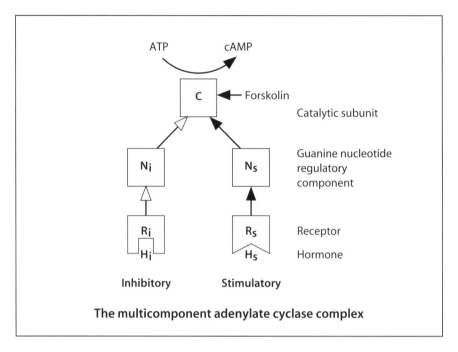

The multicomponent adenylate cyclase complex

- Inhibition of membrane transport and channel proteins.
- Stimulation of lipolysis in adipocytes.[2]
- Inhibition of glucose uptake by adipocytes, due to the binding of forskolin to glucose transport protein.[3]
- Inhibition of platelet aggregation.[4]
- Inhibition of the generation of hydroxyl radicals by platelets.[5]
- Stimulation of thyroid function with increase in thyroid hormone production.[6] However, low concentrations of forskolin may inhibit thyroid function.[7]
- Potentiation of the secretagogue effects of glucose[8] and stimulation of the release of somatostatin and glucagon.[9]
- Stimulation of ACTH, prolactin, growth hormone[10] and possibly other anterior pituitary hormones.[11]
- Enhanced secretion of acid and pepsinogen from the gastric mucosa.[12]
- Bronchodilatation.[13]
- Stimulation of maturation of follicle-enclosed oocyctes.[14]
- Stimulation of salivary, lacrimal and pancreatic glands.[15,16]
- A positive inotropic effect on the heart without increasing myocardial oxygen consumption.[17,18]

- Reduced preload and afterload of the heart due to vasodilation.[18]
- Relaxation of arteriolar smooth muscle and lowering of blood pressure.[19]
- Stimulation of steroid hormone production by adrenal and gonadal cells.[10]
- Reduction of intraocular pressure (particularly by topical application).[10]
- Cerebral vasodilation.[20]
- Inhibition of mast cell degranulation.[21]
- Inhibition of B-cell maturation.[22]
- Inhibition of mitosis of animal epidermis, indicating a possible application in psoriasis.
- Stimulation of liver glycogenolysis and gluconeogenesis.
- Possible inhibition of cancer metastasis.[23]
- Acts synergistically with calcitonin in inhibiting osteoclast function.[24]
- Acts synergistically with Crataegus which in turn is thought to inhibit phosphodiesterase,[25] the enzyme which breaks down cAMP. Combined use of Coleus and Crataegus should see cAMP levels raised through both stimulation of production and inhibition of decomposition, respectively.
- Responses to forskolin were found to be reduced in muscle cells from failing heart,[26] but since forskolin also raises cAMP, Coleus may be of benefit in this disorder.

Clinical Studies

Clinical studies are limited, although forskolin appears to have the most potential in congestive heart failure, asthma, glaucoma and as an antiplatelet agent.

- Human studies confirmed that forskolin lowers intraocular pressure by reducing the flow of aqueous humour.[27] In India, its clinical value in glaucoma was confirmed.
- Initial studies on patients with congestive cardiomyopathy and coronary artery disease confirmed that forskolin improved cardiac function and myocardial contractility.[28] A recent study found no increase in myocardial contractility at the tested dose, but left ventricular function was improved. While higher doses of forskolin did increase myocardial contractility, the accompanying large reduction in blood pressure may preclude such doses in congestive heart failure.[29]
- Clinical studies have demonstrated a bronchodilating effect in extrinsic asthmatics following chemically-induced bronchoconstriction.[30] Forskolin was inhaled and by this route was free of side-effects although its action was short-

lived. It also countered chemically-induced bronchoconstriction in a double-blind trial on healthy humans.[15]

Actions

Hypotensive, antiglaucoma, antiplatelet, bronchospasmolytic, cardiotonic.

Medicinal Uses of Coleus

- The impressive and diverse pharmacological properties of forskolin are not necessarily all relevant to herbal therapy using *Coleus forskohlii*.[31]
- Hypertension.
- Congestive heart failure, cerebrovascular disease (vasodilation) — but not to be used in cases of low blood pressure.
- Ischaemic heart disease and thrombosis (antiplatelet effect).
- Glaucoma (topically and possibly internally).
- Asthma, chronic obstructive airways disease (bronchodilatation).
- Digestive insufficiency.
- Possible uses for weight loss, psoriasis, poor fertility, mild hypothyroidism.

Combinations

Coleus can be combined with:

- Crataegus, Astragalus, *Panax ginseng* and/or Convallaria for mild congestive heart failure.
- Ephedra and/or Lobelia for bronchoconstriction.
- Zingiber and/or Curcuma (Turmeric) for antiplatelet action.
- Gentiana for stimulation of upper digestive function.
- Crataegus and/or *Salvia miltiorrhiza* for compromised cardiac function in ischaemic heart disease.
- *Ginkgo biloba* for cerebrovascular disease.
- Crataegus for hypertension.

Contraindications and Cautions

Forskolin has the ability to potentiate many drugs. Use cautiously in patients taking prescribed medication. Contraindicated in hypotension.

Dosage

6 to 12 g/day of the dried root or 6 to 12 mL of a 1:1 fluid extract. For glaucoma about 4 to 8 drops of 1:1 extract in an eye bath.

REFERENCES

1   Seamon, K B and Daly, J W: *J Cyclic Nucleotide Res* **7**, 201 (1981)

2   Ho, R J and Shi, Q H: *Biochem Biophys Res Comm* **107**, 157 (1982)

3   Laurenza, A et al: *TiPS* **10**, 442 (1989)

4   Siegl, A M et al: *Mol Pharmacol* **21**, 680 (1982)

5   Kitagawa, S: *Yakugaku Zasshi* **114**, 448, (1994)

6   Laurberg, P: *FEBS Lett* **170**, 237 (1984)

7   Brandi, M L. et al: *Acta Endocrinol* **107**, 225 (1984)

8   Henquin, J C and Meissner, H P : *Endocrinology* **115**, 1125 (1984)

9   Hermansen, K: *ibid* **116**, 2251 (1985)

10 Seamon, K B and Daly, J W in *Advances in Cyclic Nucleotide and Protein Phosphorylation Research*, Vol 20, Greengard, P and Robison, G A eds, p1, Raven Press, New York (1989)

11 Kim, K and Ramirez, V D: *Brain Research* **386**, 256 (1986)

12 Hersey, S J et al: *Biochim Biophys Acta,* **802**, 209 (1984)

13 Burka, J F: *J Pharmacol Exp Ther* **225**, 427 (1983)

14 Dekel, N and Sherizly, I: *FEBS Lett* **151**, 153 (1983)

15 Watson, E L and Dowd, F J : *Biochem Biophys Res Comm* **111**, 21 (1983)

16 Willems, P et al: *Biochim Biophys Acta* **802**, 209 (1984)

17 Metzger, H and Lindner, E: *Arzneim-Forsch* **31**, 1248 (1981)

18 de Souza, N J and Shah, V in *Economic and Medicinal Plant Research*, Vol 2, Wagner, H et al (eds), Academic Press, London (1988)

19 deSouza, N J et al: *Med Res Rev* **3**, 201 (1983)

20 Wysham, D G et al: *Stroke* **17**, 1299 (1986)

21 Marone, G et al: *Biochemical Pharmacol* **36**, 13 (1987)

22 Holte, H et al: *Eur J Immunol* **18**, 1359 (1988)

23 Agarwal, K C and Parks Jr, R E; *Int J Cancer* **32**, 801 (1983)

24 Nicholson, G C et al: *J Bone Min Res* **3**, 181 (1988)

25 Hänsel, R and Haas, H: *Therapie mit Phytopharmaka*, Springer-Verlag, Berlin (1984)

26 Harding, S E et al: *European Heart Journal* **15** suppl D, 35 (1994)

27 Burstein, N L et al: *Exp Eye Res* **39**, 745 (1984)

28 Linderer, T and Biamino, G in *Forskolin: Its Chemical, Biological and Medical Potential*, Rupp, R H et al (eds), pp 109 to 113, Hoechst India Ltd., Bombay (1986)

29 Kramer, W et al: *Arzneim-Forsch* **37**, 364 (1987)

30 Lichey, J et al: *Lancet* **2**, 167 (1984)

31 Bone, K: *The Curious Case of Coleus*, MediHerb Professional Newsletter, December (1990)

Commiphora mukul

Sanskrit	Guggula
English	Gum guggul, Guggul
Family	Burseracae
Part Used	Resinous exudate

An oleo-gum-resin similar to Myrrh, yellowish in colour. A well-known Ayurvedic herb for the treatment of arthritis which has recently come into prominence as an effective treatment for high blood cholesterol. Initial investigations were inspired by an ancient Sanskrit text which pointed to Guggul as a treatment for obesity and associated lipid disorders.

Active Constituents

Are probably a mixture of lipid-soluble steroids found in the resin including guggulsterones E and Z.[1]

Guggulsterone E   Guggulsterone Z

Pharmacology

➜ *Cholesterol Lowering Effects*

- Preliminary studies showed that Guggul prevented hypercholesterolaemia and atheroma in cholesterol-fed rabbits.[2]
- This was followed up by similar studies in chicks, rats, pigs and gerbils.[2]

- Oral administration of the ethylacetate extract of *C. mukul* significantly prevented the rise in serum cholesterol and triglycerides in rats caused by an atherogenic diet.[3]

- Attempts have been made to understand the mechanism of the cholesterol-lowering effect. These include:

  - Demonstration of a strong thyroid-stimulating activity for Z guggulsterone in rats at 10 mg/kg.[6] The thyroid-stimulating effect is different from that of TSH (thyroid stimulating hormone and is probably not mediated through the pituitary. Z guggulsterone probably has a direct effect on the thyroid gland.[4,5] (Thyroid stimulation reduces serum cholesterol.

  - Stimulation of LDL receptor activity in the liver membrane causing enhanced uptake of LDL and decreased cholesterol biosynthesis.[6]

➜ *Anti-inflammatory Activity*

- Guggul is traditionally also used for arthritis and its anti-inflammatory activity has been confirmed.[7]

- The aqueous extract of *C. mukul* was also found to exert an anti-inflammatory effect by inhibiting oedema in carrageenin-induced rat paw oedema.[8]

➜ *Other Effects*

- Studies on haematological parameters in animals and humans have also shown:[2,9]

  - Increased coagulation and prothrombin time.

  - Decreased platelet adhesiveness.

  - Increased fibrinolytic activity.

  - Inhibition of platelet aggregation by the guggulsterones.

- In chemically induced myocardial necrosis, guggulsterones reversed metabolic changes that may lead to formation of free radicals.[10] A protective effect on cardiac enzymes and the cytochrome P-450 system was also observed.[11]

Clinical Studies

➜ *Cholesterol Lowering Effects*

- Many clinical trials have been conducted.[2] Two controlled trials used a semi-refined, ethyl acetate extract of the gum (gugulipid) to reduce side effects. In these trials a placebo was used for a similar or shorter period. Results were as follows:

- 77% of patients responded to treatment over 12 weeks and the average decreases in responders were 17.5% for serum cholesterol and 30.3% for serum triglycerides.[12]
- 59% of patients responded to treatment over 6 weeks and the average decreases in responders were 24.5% for serum cholesterol and 27.3% for serum triglycerides.[13]

- In a randomised double blind trial, 31 patients were given 100 mg per day of gugulipid over 6 months, and 30 patients received a placebo.[14] In addition these patients and controls received a fruit and vegetable enriched diet. The following results were observed:
  - total cholesterol decreased by 11.7%.
  - LDL-cholesterol decreased by 12.5%.
  - triglycerides decreased by 12%.
  - total cholesterol/HDL-cholesterol decreased by 11.1%.
  - an antioxidant effect as indicated by decreased lipid peroxide levels (by 33.3%).
  - Side effects were observed in a few patients (headache, mild nausea, eructation and hiccough.[14]

- A double blind cross-over trial was conducted on 125 hyperlipidaemic patients in several clinics across India. The trial compared the effect of gugulipid to the drug clofibrate. Patients received 1000 mg per day of gugulipid over a period of 12 weeks.
  - In patients treated with gugulipid serum cholesterol was reduced by 12.6% and serum triglycerides by 16.4% on average.
  - In hypercholesterolaemic patients the response with gugulipid was better but clofibrate showed a better response in patients with hypertriglyceridaemia. Response to both drugs was comparable in mixed hyperlipidaemic patients.
  - HDL-cholesterol was significantly increased only in those who received gugulipid.
  - A reduction in the ratio of LDL-cholesterol / HDL-cholesterol and total cholesterol / HDL-cholesterol was observed more with gugulipid than with clofibrate in 45 patients.[15]

➡ *Other Conditions*

- A progressive reduction in lesions in a majority of 10 patients with nodulocystic acne was observed following treatment with a gugulipid tablet (equivalent to 25 mg guggulsterone) twice daily for 3 months. Only 2 of the patients suffered relapse after 3 months. Compared to tetracycline, patients with oily skin were observed to respond better to gugulipid.[16]

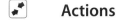

Actions

Anticholesterolaemic, antiplatelet, anti-inflammatory, antiobesity.

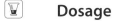

Medicinal Uses

- High blood cholesterol and triglycerides.
- Arthritis.
- Ischaemic heart disease (see *Inula racemosa*).
- Older texts cite its value in weight loss and this was evident in some trials.
- Acne.

Dosage

1200 to 1500 mg/day of the extract (gugulipid) corresponding to approximately 48-60 mg/day of guggulsterones. Do not give during breast-feeding.

REFERENCES

1 Patil, V D et al: *Tetrahedron* **28**, 2341 (1972)
2 Satyavati, G V: *Indian J Med Res* **87**, 327 (1988)
3 Lata, S et al: *J Postgraduate Medicine* **37**, 132 (1991)
4 Tripathi, Y B et al: *Planta Medica* p78, (1984)
5 Tripathi, Y B et al: *Planta Medica* p271 (1988)
6 Singh, V et al: *Pharmacol Res* **22**, 37 (1990)
7 Sharma, J N et al: *Arzneim-Forsch* **27**, 1455 (1977)
8 Duwiejua, M et al: *Planta Medica* **59**, 12 (1993)
9 Mester, L et al: *Planta Medica* **37**, 367 (1979)
10 Kaul, S et al: *Indian J Exp Biol* **27**, 625 (1989)
11 Kaul, S et al: *Indian J Exp Biol* **90**, 62 (1989)
12 Agarwal, R C et al: *Indian J Med Res* **84**, 626 (1986)
13 Gopal, K et al: *J Assoc Physicians India* **34**, 249 (1986)
14 Singh, R B et al: *Cardio Drugs Therapy* **8**, 659 (1994)
15 Nityanand, S et al: J Assoc Phys Ind **37**, 323 (1989)
16 Thappa, D M et al: *J Dermatology* **21**, 729 (1994)

Crataeva nurvala

Sanskrit	Varuna
English	The Three-leaved Caper
Family	Capparidaceae
Parts Used	Bark or root bark

Cultivated in the vicinity of temples in Central India.

Active Constituents

Contains saponins, flavonoids, glucosinolates,[1] tannins and plant sterols (lupeol).[2]

Lupeol

Pharmacology

- Increases tone of smooth and skeletal muscle *in vitro*.[3]
- The petroleum ether extract was shown to inhibit acute and chronic inflammation.[4]
- Decreases bladder-stone formation in an experimental model in rats.[5] The weight of the stone in the treated group was significantly less than the control group. The bladders of treated animals showed less oedema, ulceration and cellular infiltration when compared to controls.

- Oral treatment for 40 days increased bladder tone in dogs.[5]
- Decreased tendency to form calcium oxalate kidney stones was observed in rats treated with Crataeva decoction.[6]
- Oral administration of lupeol, a plant steroid isolated from Crataeva, inhibited stone formation in rats, exhibited stone-dissolving activity and facilitated the passage of very small calculi from the bladder. Altered levels of urea and creatinine, which were indicative of kidney dysfunction, were also restored to normal.[7]
- Oral doses of an alcoholic extract of Crataeva also demonstrated significant dose-dependent preventative activity against experimental urolith formation in rats.[8] Crataeva also reversed biochemical parameters associated with urolith formation towards normal levels.[8]

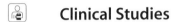

Clinical Studies

➜ Bladder Tone

- Decoction of Crataeva was tested on 30 patients with hypotonic bladder due to benign prostatic hyperplasia.[5] There was marked relief of frequency, incontinence, pain and retention of urine. Urine flow improved and there was an increase in bladder tone after therapy. Improvement in the symptoms of persistent hypotonia, atony and neurogenic bladder were also observed, with residual volume of urine decreased and bladder tone improved after application of Crataeva.[5]

➜ Urinary Tract Stones

- After treatment with Crataeva decoction, the urine of patients became less lithogenic.[5] Urinary calcium was reduced and urinary sodium and magnesium increased significantly.[5] A pharmacological study found that Crataeva influenced small intestinal (Na^+,K^+)-ATPases which may in turn influence the transport of minerals.[9]
- A clinical study of the effects of Crataeva decoction on 46 patients with kidney, ureter or bladder stones not requiring surgery found 26 patients passed the stones within 10 weeks of treatment. The majority of the remaining patients experienced symptom relief.[5]

➜ Urinary Tract Infections

- A majority (85%) of patients with proven chronic urinary tract infections were symptom-free after 4 weeks' treatment with Crataeva decoction.[5] There was no data for controls.

Actions

Antilithic, bladder tonic, anti-inflammatory.

 ## Medicinal Uses

- Chronic urinary tract infections in conjunction with antiseptics and immuno-stimulants.
- Prevention and treatment of kidney stones.
- Benign prostatic hyperplasia in combination with Pygeum.
- Hypotonic and atonic bladder.
- Incontinence and possibly enuresis.
- The foremost Ayurvedic herb for the urinary tract.

 ## Dosage

Best results are obtained following administration of 15 to 25 g/day as a decoction of the dried bark or root bark. Otherwise 5 to 10 mL per day of the 1:2 extract.

REFERENCES

1   Sharma, V and Padhya, M A: *Indian Drugs* **26**, 572 (1989)
2   Prabhakar, Y S and Kumar, D S: *Fitoterapia* **61**, 99 (1990)
3   Prasad, D N et al: *J Res Ind Med* **1**, 120 (1966)
4   Das, P K et al: *ibid* **9**, 49 (1974)
5   Deshpande, P J et al: *Indian J Med Res* **76**, 46 (1982)
6   Varalakshmi, P et al: *J Ethnopharmacol* **28**, 313 (1990)
7   Anand, R et al: *Proc 24th Indian Pharmacol Soc Conf,* Ahmedabad, Gujarat, India A10, Dec 29 to 31, (1991)
8   Anand, R et al: *Fitoterapia* **64**, 345 (1993)
9   Varalakshmi, P et al: *J Ethnopharmacol* **31**, 67 (1991)

Gymnema sylvestre

Hindi	Gurmar — "sugar destroyer"
English	Small Indian Ipecac
Family	Asclepiadaceae
Part Used	Leaves

A stout, large, woody, climbing plant which grows in Central and Southern India. Is also a native of tropical Australia although other Gymnema species are more abundant there.

Active Constituents

Gymnemic acids — a chemically complex mixture of saponins. Gurmarin — a polypeptide of 35 amino acids.

Pharmacology

- Leaves thought to increase insulin secretion.[1]

- Early studies showed no significant effect on blood sugar levels in normal rats, but there was a significant reduction for rats made hyperglycaemic by various means. Decreased body weight was also countered.

- Gymnema regulated blood sugar levels in alloxan diabetic rabbits and increased activities of the enzymes which facilitate use of glucose by insulin-dependent pathways. Uptake of glucose into glycogen and protein was increased in liver, kidney and muscle.[2]

- Gymnema corrected the hyperglycaemia in mild alloxan diabetic rats and prolonged life-span in severe alloxan diabetic rats.[3]

- Gymnema extract and gymnemic acid significantly depressed the portal release of gastric inhibitory peptide after intraduodenal glucose infusion. They may be interacting with a glucose receptor which exists for the release of gastric inhibitory peptide.[4]

- The gymnemic acids are considered to be the antisweet principles,[5] but a peptide (gurmarin) has also been isolated with significant antisweet activity.[6]

- Two recent pharmacological studies have provided clear evidence for the benefits of Gymnema in diabetic models. In a Japanese study on mildly diabetic rats, 28 days of Gymnema use reduced post-prandial serum glucose and improved glucose tolerance. Pancreas weight and content of insulin were not changed.[7]

- In contrast, an Indian study found that Gymnema extract returned fasting blood glucose levels to normal in diabetic rats after twenty days of oral administration. Therapy led to a rise in insulin, and pancreatic islet regeneration occurred to some extent.[8]

Clinical Studies

- Two long-term Indian studies without placebo controls yielded promising results in diabetic patients. The first study on insulin-dependent diabetes mellitus found that Gymnema extract reduced insulin requirements and fasting blood glucose, glycosylated haemoglobin and glycosylated plasma protein levels. There was some suggestion of enhancement of endogenous insulin production, possibly by pancreatic regeneration.[1]

- The second study by the same research group on non-insulin-dependent diabetics found Gymnema extract produced similar results to the above study and hypoglycaemic drug requirements were reduced. Fasting and post-prandial serum insulin levels were elevated in the Gymnema group compared to controls taking only conventional drugs.[1]

- Clinical research under double blind conditions found that gymnemic acid considerably diminished the sweet taste. However, the study also revealed that gymnemic acid also significantly decreased appetite for up to 90 minutes after the sweet-numbing effect.[9]

Other Applications

- Gymnema anaesthetises the sweet taste buds, an effect which can last many hours. This may have implications, both subtle and obvious, in weight control and dieting.[9]

- May be useful for athletes in developing a higher ratio of muscle mass to body fat because of the increased insulin output with long-term use.

Actions

Hypoglycaemic, antidiabetic, hypocholesterolaemic.

Medicinal Uses

- Some cases of diabetes will respond quickly but best results come after six to twelve months of continuous use.

- To reduce sweet craving and appetite.

Dosage

5 to 10 mL/day of the 1:1 extract for diabetes. Less may be needed if combined with other antidiabetic herbs. Only 1 to 2 mL per day is necessary for sweet-craving and sweet taste depression. In the latter case the drops should be applied directly to the tongue and rinsed off after one minute. This can be done at two to three hour intervals.

REFERENCES

1   Shanmugasundaram, E R et al: *J Ethnopharmacol* **30**, 281 and 295 (1990)

2   Shanmugasundaram, K R et al: *J Ethnopharmacol* **7**, 205 (1983)

3   Srivastava, Y et al: *Int J Crude Drug Res* **24**, 171 (1986)

4   Fushiki, T et al: *J Nutr* **122**, 2367 (1992)

5   Liu, H M et al: *Chem Pharm Bull (Tokyo)* **40**, 1366 (1992)

6   Imoto, T et al: *Comp Biochem Physiol* **100**, 309 (1991)

7   Okabayashi, Y et al: *Diabetes Res Clin Pract* **9**, 143 (1990)

8   Baskaran, K et al: *J Ethnopharmacol* **30**, 265 (1990)

9   Brala, P M and Hagen, R L : *Physiology and Behaviour* **30**, 1 (1983)

Hemidesmus indicus

Sanskrit	Anantamul
English	Indian Sarsaparilla
Family	Asclepiadaceae
Part Used	Root

A climbing vine found throughout India.

Active Constituents

Coumarin, essential oil, triterpenoid saponins.

Pharmacology

- As Hemidesmus contains significant amounts of coumarin, it will have similar actions to Melilotus.

- Hemidesmus has been found to depress both the cell-mediated and humoral components of the immune system.[1]

- An inhibiting effect on leprosy was found in mice foot-pads[2] which is probably due to an antimicrobial effect.

- An organic acid isolated from the root of Hemidesmus demonstrated viper venom inhibitory activity in rodents.[3] The lethal haemorrhagic, coagulant and anticoagulant activity induced by the viper venom was inhibited by the acid.

Actions

Depurative, diaphoretic, immunosuppressant.

Medicinal Uses

- Chronic skin diseases and ulcers.
- Autoimmune disease e.g. rheumatoid arthritis.
- Although mildly immunosuppressant, is very safe and non-toxic.
- Often combined with Picrorrhiza.

Dosage

3 to 6 mL per day of the 1:2 extract.

REFERENCES

1   Atal, C.K et al: *J Ethnopharmacol* **18**, 133 (1986)
2   Gupta, P.N: *Lepr India* **53**, 354 (1981)
3   Alam, M I et al: *Toxicon* **32**, 1551 (1994)

Inula racemosa

A close relative of Elecampane.

Sanskrit	Pushkarmoola
Family	Asteraceae
Part Used	Root

Pushkarmoola is traditionally used for cough, dyspnoea and chest (precordial) pain. It has also been extensively used for heart disease.

Active Constituents

Sesquiterpene lactones, such as alantolactone, isoalantolactone, inunal and iso-alloalantolactone,[1] essential oil.

Alantolactone   **Inunal**

Pharmacology

- Animal experiments have shown spasmolytic effects on uterine and ileal smooth muscle.[2]

- Inula protects against bronchospasm induced by histamine, serotonin and pollens.[2]

Clinical Studies

- *Inula racemosa* prevented ECG signs of ischaemia after exercise in patients with ischaemic heart disease. Results were comparable to or greater than glyceryl trinitrate and more long-lived. Follow-up pharmacological studies suggested a beta-blocking type of action.[3]

- A combination of *Inula racemosa* and *Commiphora mukul* has been extensively studied in ischaemic heart disease. The dose was 6 g/day over 4 months in 50 patients. Precordial pain, dyspnoea and discomfort were controlled or improved in 90% of patients and cholesterol decreased by 17%. Objective ECG analysis showed marked improvement in 30% of cases (many patients had irreversible changes due to ischaemic damage).[4]

- *Inula racemosa* was found to possess significant antianginal activity in an open clinical study on 30 patients with angina pectoris. It lowered diastolic blood pressure, plasma cortisol and catecholamines.[5]

Adverse Effects

Alantolactone has been shown to demonstrate a sensitizing capacity in mice investigated for allergic contact dermatitis.[6]

Actions

Antispasmodic, beta-blocking, hypotensive, antianginal.

Medicinal Uses

- Ischaemic heart disease, angina.
- Bronchial disease and asthma.
- Specifically indicated for chronic bronchitis with cardiac complications.

Dosage

2 to 4 g/day of the dried root or 4 to 8 mL/day of the 1:2 extract.

REFERENCES

1   Kalsi, P S et al: *Phytochemistry* **27**, 2079 (1988)
2   Singh, N et al: *Quart J Crude Drug Res* **18**, 89 (1980)
3   Tripathi, Y B et al: *J Ethnopharmacology* **23**, 3 (1988)
4   Tripathi, S N et al: *Ancient Science of Life* **4**, 9 (1984)
5   Dwivedi, S et al: *Int J Crude Drug Res* **27**, 217 (1989)
6   Alonso Blasi N et al: *Arch Derm Res* **284**, 297 (1992)

Phyllanthus amarus

Also known as *Phyllanthus niruri* (see below).

Sanskrit	Bahupatra
Family	Euphorbiaceae
Parts Used	Leaves or aerial parts

This is an important traditional remedy in the south of India for the treatment of jaundice. It has recently come into prominence among Western scientists due to a clinical trial published in *The Lancet*.[1]

Active Constituents

Lignans such as phyllanthin and hypophyllanthin,[2] flavonoids and alkaloids, and the *in vitro* antiviral agent geraniin, which is a tannin.[3]

Pharmacology

Although *P. niruri* is often used to denote *P. amarus*, it is actually endemic to West Indies and not found in India. *P. niruri* is represented by 3 different species: *P. amarus*, *P. fraterus* and *P. debilis*. Much of the work previously carried out in India on plants called *P. niruri* was done on these other species.[4]

→ *Antiviral Activity*

- The herb causes *in vitro* inactivation of HBsAg (hepatitis B surface antigen).[5]
- Phyllanthus inhibits hepatitis B virus (HBV) and binds to its surface antigen *in vitro*.[6] The hepatitis B virus requires DNA polymerase for its replication, and the action of Phyllanthus in inhibiting this enzyme appears to be specific to HBV-like viruses.[6]
- Chemical fractions of *Phyllanthus amarus* extract were effective against HBV antigens *in vitro*, and inhibited the interaction of HBsAg and hepatitis B envelope antigen (HBeAg) with their corresponding antibodies.[7]
- Phyllanthus decreases the titre of woodchuck hepatitis virus surface antigen faster than controls. Some animals became and remained free of the virus marker.[6]

- The plant is certainly active *in vitro*, but its *in vivo* activity has been questioned in recent studies. So while recent studies have shown that Phyllanthus can suppress the HBsAg gene expression in human hepatoma cells and can bind to HBV antigens,[8] the herb failed to inhibit viral replication in ducks, although duck HBsAg levels were reduced in some cases.[9]

- No definite antiviral activity was observed in 114 ducks infected with duck HBV treated with *P. amarus* and *P. maderaspatensis*.[10] Five Australian Phyllanthus species were found to cause 50% inhibition at concentrations of 350–800 mg/mL duck HBV *in vitro*.[11] These extracts did not prevent or eliminate infections when adminstered *in vivo*.[11]

- Aqueous extract of Phyllanthus inhibited human immunodeficiency virus (HIV) reverse transcriptase *in vitro*. The component responsible for the inhibition was identified as repandusinic acid A.[12]

➜ **Hepatoprotective Activity**

- The lignans show a mild hepatoprotective activity for *in vitro* tests.[2]

➜ **Other Effects**

- The increased fatty deposition in the liver, brain, kidney and heart of rats after ethanol administration was normalised by a dose of 200mg/rat/day.[13]

- Phyllanthus extract lowers blood glucose in diabetic rats.[14]

- The lignans phyllanthin and hypophyllanthin were found to enhance the cytotoxic response cause by vinblastine on cultured multi-drug-resistant cells.[15]

Clinical Studies

- In children with jaundice due to viral hepatitis, a dose of 50 mg/kg caused rapid improvement in most cases. However results were not conclusive due to the lack of controls.[16]

- *The Lancet* Study (Thyagarajan et al):[1]
  - Dose was 600 mg/day of leaf.
  - Study was on carriers of hepatitis B virus.
  - 59% of 37 treated subjects compared to only 4% of placebo subjects had lost HBsAg by the first follow up visit (15 to 20 days).
  - Up to nine months later HBsAg had not returned for these subjects.
  - There were no significant side effects.
  - Results are only preliminary since HBsAg is not the only marker and HBeAg is more indicative of loss of replicating virus from the system. In fact

HBsAg-positive carriers with HBeAg were found to be less likely to respond to treatment.

- Many clinical studies which followed have been negative. A Thai,[17] an Indian,[18] and a Dutch study using Phyllanthus from Suriname[19] all found that no significant loss of HBsAg occurred.

- A mildly positive study, also from Thailand, noted some loss of HBsAg in the treated group. However in most of the above negative studies, Indian grown plant was not used and it is possible that the Indian variety is more potent.[20]

- A recent New Zealand study (Milne et al) using a standardized extract of *P. amarus* (20 mg geraniin per dose) also failed to confirm the Lancet study.[3] No effect on HBsAg or HBeAg levels were observed in patients given 3 doses per day for 2 months.

- The authors suggest that the conflicting outcomes of previous trials may be due to the use of plants from many different areas.

- Milne reports that when the authors of the Lancet study (Thyagarajan et al[1]) repeated their trial, the success rate was only 20%.[3] However, this success rate is still better than that found by other groups.

- In conclusion, Phyllanthus sourced from India may have a role in viral liver diseases (as maintained by tradition), but it should be used in combination with other treatments.

Actions

Antiviral, hepatoprotective, hypoglycaemic.

Medicinal Uses

- Viral liver diseases, including acute hepatitis and chronic persistent hepatitis. As part of the treatment for chronic active hepatitis.

- Possibly other viral diseases.

- May have a support role in diabetes.

Dosage

2 to 6 mL/day of the 1:2 extract. Higher end of the dosage range for acute states.

REFERENCES

1   Thyagarajan, S P et al: *Lancet* **2**, 764 (1988)
2   Syamasundar, K V et al: *J Ethnopharmacol* **14**, 41 (1985)
3   Milne, A et al: *New Zeal Med J* **107**, 243 (1994)
4   Bagchi, G D et al: *Int J Pharmacog* **30**, 161 (1992)

5   Thyagarajan, S P et al: *Indian J Med Res* **76**, 124 (1982)

6   Venkateswaran, P S et al: *Proc Natl Acad Sci USA* **84**, 274 (1987)

7   Mehrotra, R et al: *Indian J Med Res* **93**, 71 (1991)

8   Yeh, S F et al: *Antiviral Res* **20**, 185 (1993)

9   Nui, J et al: *J Med Virol* **32**, 212 (1990)

10   Munshi, A et al: *J Med Virol* **40**, 275 (1993)

11   Shead, A et al: *Antiviral Res* **18**, 127 (1992)

12   Ogata, T et al: *AIDS Res Hum Retroviruses* **8**, 1937 (1992)

13   Umarani, D et al: *Ancient Sci Life* **4**, 174 (1985)

14   Higashino, H et al: *Nippon Yakurigaku Zasshi* **100**, 415 (1992)

15   Somanabandhu, A et al: *J Nat Prod* **56**, 233 (1993)

16   Dixit, S P and Achar, M P: *J Natl Integ Med Assoc* **25**, 269 (1983)

17   Leelarasamee, A et al: *Lancet* **335**, 1600 (1990)

18   Doshi, J C et al: *Indian J Gastroenterol* **13**, 7 (1994)

19   Berk, L et al: *J Hepatology* **12**, 405 (1991)

20   Thamlikitkul, V et al: *J Med Assoc Thai* **74**, 381 (1991)

Picrorrhiza kurroa

Sanskrit	Katuka
Family	Scrophulariaceae
Part Used	Root

A small herb which grows in the Himalayas at 3000 to 5000m.

Active Constituents

Iridoid glycosides such as picrosides I, II, III and kutkoside. More recently nine cucurbitacin glycosides (highly oxygenated triterpenes) have been identified which would explain the exceptional bitterness of the root (six of these are illustrated below). Other active compounds include apocynin and androsin.[1-5]

Cucurbitacin glycosides

R¹	R²	R³	Other
O=	O=	OAc	$\Delta^{23,24}$
O=	O=	OAc	–
HO	H₂	OAc	$\Delta^{23,24}$
HO	H₂	OH	$\Delta^{23,24}$
HO	H₂	OH	–
HO	O=	OAc	$\Delta^{23,24}$

Picroside I

Pharmacology

➜ Hepatoprotective Activity

- A potent hepatoprotective action for Picrorrhiza and its components has been demonstrated against a variety of toxins.[6–20] The activity of Picroliv (a standardised extract containing a total of 60% picroside I and kutkoside) was found in many of these tests to be comparable on superior to silymarin from *Silybum marianum*.

- A study on rat liver tissue found Picrorrhiza restored (Na^+, K^+)-ATPase activity after chemical damage. Free radical scavenging activity was observed *in vitro* by the use of Picroliv. Oral doses were found to stimulate nucleic acid and protein synthesis in rat liver.[21–23]

- Picrorrhiza and its components showed marked activity against human hepatitis B surface antigen *in vitro*. Its action was stronger than silymarin.[24] Picroside I and II demonstrated preventative activity *in vitro* against immune-mediated liver damage.[25] The activity was comparable to silybin from *Silybum marianum*. However, the cucurbitacins may slightly accentuate hepatotoxicity.[25]

➜ Choleretic Activity

- Picroliv exhibited a dose-dependent choleretic effect in rats and guinea-pigs. Increases in bile flow, bile salt and bile acid output were observed.[12]

➜ Antioxidant Activity

- Antioxidant activity was observed after oral doses *in vivo*. Reduction of lipid peroxidation within microsomes by Picroliv was also observed *in vitro*.[26]

➜ Bronchial Effects

- Picrorrhiza had a greater effect than disodium cromoglycate in reducing bronchial allergic reaction in guinea pigs.[27] Mast cell stabilization was observed following the use of Picrorrhiza *in vivo*.[28]

- Oral doses of androsin (a component of Picrorrhiza) inhibited allergen- and PAF-induced bronchial obstruction, but had no bronchodilating activity.[29]

➜ Anti-inflammatory Activity

- The water-soluble fraction of the alcoholic extract of Picrorrhiza demonstrated an anti-inflammatory effect mediated through increased sensitivity of β-adrenergic receptors and impairment of pro-inflammatory cells.[30,31] There was no effect on prostaglandin production.

- Apocynin (a catechol in Picrorrhiza) was found to be an effective and selective inhibitor of neutrophil oxidative burst *in vitro*.[32] Oral administration to animals produced a significant reduction in joint swelling in immune-mediated arthritis.[33] There was no evidence of rebound flare-up of joint swelling after the treatment was stopped.

- Apocynin is believed to inhibit thromboxane synthetase and with it, arachidonic-acid-induced platelet aggregation.[34] This suggests an antiplatelet activity in addition to the anti-inflammatory activity.

➜ Immunologic Function

- Oral doses of Picrorrhiza extract significantly boosted T-cell, B-cell and phagocytic function in rats.[36]
- Oral administration of Picroliv at 10 mg/kg for 7 days enhanced a broad range of antigen-specific and non-specific immune responses, including significant protection against *Leishmania donovani* infection.[37]

➜ Other Activity

- The effect of Picroliv was evaluated on potentiation of the antifilarial activity of a drug in rats infected with a filarial strain. Although Picroliv did not exert any effect on adult parasites, in combination with ivermectin it exerted a significant lethal effect on macrofilariids.[38]

Clinical Studies

➜ Hepatitis

- Clinical trials using Picrorrhiza for the treatment of infective hepatitis demonstrated rapid falls in bilirubin levels and quicker clinical recovery.[39,40]

➜ Asthma

- A poorly-designed study failed to demonstrated a significant result for asthma although there was a trend to clinical improvement.[39]
- In an uncontrolled study using 400 mg/day of Picrorrhiza root, marked relief was observed in all of 25 cases of asthma.[41] Remission of rheumatic pains was also observed in 4 cases. Open trials on osteoarthritis, ankylosing spondylitis, psoriasis and vitiligo showed a favourable response.[41]

➜ Other Conditions

- A 7-year controlled clinical trial using 400 mg per day of Picrorrhiza root on patients with vitiligo revealed marked benefits when Picrorrhiza was combined with photochemotherapy.[36]

Adverse Effects

High doses may cause diarrhoea, flatulence and griping (cucurbitacins) in sensitive individuals. Picrorrhiza also can cause a skin rash. Some patients find the bitterness intolerable.

Actions

Hepatoprotective, anti-inflammatory, antiallergic, immunostimulator, bitter tonic, choleretic.

Medicinal Uses

- Acute and chronic infections, weakened immunity.
- As adjuvant therapy in allergies and autoimmune disorders.
- Toxic liver damage, liver infections.
- Asthma

Dosage

500 mg to 2g/day of the dried root or 1 to 4 mL/day of 1:2 extract.

REFERENCES

1   Weinges, K et al: *Liebigs Ann Chem* **759**, 173 (1972)
2   Singh, B and Rastogi, R P: *Ind J Chem* **10**, 29 (1972)
3   Stuppner, H and Wagner, H: *Planta Medica* **55**, 559 (1989)
4   Stuppner, H et al: *Planta Medica* **55**, 620 (1989)
5   Stuppner, H and Wagner, H: *Planta Medica* **55**, 467 (1989)
6   Pandey, V N and Chaturvedi, G N: *Ind J Med Res* **57**, 503 (1969)
7   Ansari, R A et al: *Ind J Med Res* **87**, 401 (1988)
8   Chander, R et al: *Ind J Med Res* **92**, 34 (1990)
9   Floersheim, G L et al: *Agents and Actions* **29**, 386 (1990)
10 Dwivedi, Y et al: *Planta Medica* **57**, 25 (1991)
11 Ansari, R et al: *J Ethnopharmacol* **34**, 61 (1991)
12 Shukla, B et al: *Planta Medica* **57**, 29 (1991)
13 Dwivedi, Y et al: *Chung Kuo Yao Li Hsueh Pao* **13**, 197 (1992)
14 Singh, V et al: *Ind J Biochem Biophys* **29**, 428 (1992)
15 Saraswat, B et al: *Ind J Exp Biol* **31**, 316 (1993)
16 Chander, R et al: *Ind J Exp Biol* **30**, 711 (1992)
17 Dwivedi, Y et al: *Pharmacol Res* **27**, 189 (1993)
18 Dwivedi, Y et al: *Pharmacol Toxicol* **71**, 383 (1992)
19 Visen, P K et al: *Planta Medica* **59**, 37 (1993)
20 Dwivedi, Y et al: *Pharmacol Res* **23**, 399 (1991)
21 Mogre, K et al: *Ind J Pharmac* **13**, 253 (1981)

22   Chander, R et al: *Biochem Pharm* **44**, 180 (1992)

23   Singh, V et al: *Ind J Exp Biol* **30**, 68 (1992)

24   Mehrotra, R et al: *Ind J Med Res* **92**, 133 (1990)

25   Kiso, Y et al: *Planta Medica* **53**, 241' (1987)

26   Chander, R et al: *Ind J Exp Biol* **32**, 324 (1994)

27   Mahajani, S S and Kulkarni, R D: *Int Arch Allergy Appl Immun* **53**, 137 (1977)

28   Pandey, B L and Das, P K: *Ind J Allergy Appl Immunol* **2**, 21 (1988)

29   Dorsch, W et al: *Int Arch Allergy Appl Immunol* **95**, 128 (1991)

30   Pandey, B L and Das, P K: *Ind J Physiol Pharmac* **32**, 120 (1988)

31   Pandey, B L and Das, P D: *Ind J Physiol Pharmac* **32**, 289 (1988)

32   Simons, J M et al: *Free Rad Biol Med* **8**, 251 (1990)

33   'tHart, B A et al: *Free Rad Biol Med* **9**, 127 (1990)

34   Engels, F et al: *Febs Lett* **305**, 254 (1992)

35   Puri, A et al: *Planta Medica* **58**, 528 (1992)

36   Atal, C K et al: *J Ethnopharmacol* **18**, 133 (1986)

37   Bedi, K L: *J Ethnopharmacol* **27**, 347 (1989)

38   Fatma, N et al: *Acta Tropica* **57**, 55 (1994)

39   Doshi, V B et al: *J Postgrad Med* **29**, 89 (1983)

40   Shan, B K et al: *J Postgrad Med* **23**, 188 (1977)

41   Langer, J G et al: *Ind J Pharmacol* **13**, 98 (1981)

Terminalia arjuna

Sanskrit	Arjuna
English	Arjun tree
Family	Combretaceae
Part Used	Bark

Many Terminalias are used in Ayurvedic medicine. However this tree has been prized as a treatment for heart disorders for over 3000 years. It is a tropical woody tree found throughout India near rivers and streams which grows up to 30 metres. The bark is very thick, smooth and pinkish grey.

Active Constituents

Tannins, triterpenoid saponins (arjungenin, arjunglucosides), flavonoids (arjunone, arjunolone), phytosterols.[1]

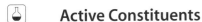

Arjunglucoside III   Arjunolone

Pharmacology

→ *Cardiovascular System*

- Conflicting results were observed with early studies showing an increase in heart rate and blood pressure. Later studies showed a dose-dependent decrease.[2]

- Terminalia is known to assist the nutrient supply to the heart, the heart muscle gains energy so that the heart beat is strong and the number of beats is reduced.[3]
- Enhancement of PGE_2-like activity after ischaemia was observed.[4]

→ **Other Effects**

- Contradictory findings were reported on coagulation in rabbits, with some studies finding no effect on prothrombin time, some reduced and others increased.[5]
- Terminalia has shown a reduction in total cholesterol and triglycerides and an elevation in HDL-cholesterol in rabbits receiving a high cholesterol diet.[6,7]
- Diuretic effects have been reported.[1]

Clinical Studies

- No effect was found in severe congestive heart failure in early studies.
- Another study found 42% improvement in congestive heart failure, 62% improvement in symptoms of hypertension (with less improvement in the actual hypertension) and 40% improvement in symptoms of cirrhosis.[1,4]
- A case study of complete heart block due to ischaemia showed dramatic improvement to sinus rhythm after 3 months.[4]
- Terminalia was found effective in alleviating anginal pain in a study on 30 patients, especially in cases with ectopic beats. It also improved risk factors such as hypertension.[4]
- A recent open study of the effects of *Terminalia arjuna* in angina patients found a 50% decrease in angina episodes ($p<0.01$) in 15 patients with stable angina pectoris.[8] Other symptoms of angina improved, including lowered systolic blood pressure and a delayed time to onset of angina. Patients with unstable angina did not show significant improvement.[8]
- The general conclusion is that Terminalia is cardioprotective, not cardiotonic.

Adverse Effects

An Indian doctor reported a patient, who after consuming Terminalia for about four years, developed acute myocardial infarction. There was no previous history of any cardiac illness except one episode of sinus tachycardia. It was suggested that cases of stable angina should be treated with Terminalia alone with extreme caution.[9] However, the findings of this single case should be balanced against the successful clinical trial cited above.[8]

Actions

Cardioprotective, hepatoprotective, mild diuretic.

Medicinal Uses

- Ischaemic heart disease, angina.
- Cardiac arrhythmias.

Dosage

1 to 3 g/day of the dried bark or 2 to 6 mL of the 1:2 extract. Higher doses for decoctions.

REFERENCES

1 Kumar, D S and Prabhaker, Y S: *J Ethnopharmacol* **20**, 173 (1987)
2 Dwivedi, S and Udupa, N: *Fitoterapia* **60**, 413, (1989)
3 Wahal, P K: *Probe* **30**, 312 (1991) in Vaidya, A B: *J Assoc Physicians Ind* **42**, 281 (1994)
4 Dwivedi, S et al: *Indian Drugs* **24**, 378 (1987)
5 Phadnaik, B S and Parasar, G C: *Punjabrao Krishi Vidyapeeth Res J* **5**, 1 (1981)
6 Tiwari, A K et al: *Int J Crude Drug Res* **28**, 43 (1990)
7 Pathak, S R et al: *Int J Crude Drug Res* **28**, 43 (1990) in Vaidya, A B: *J Assoc Physicians Ind* **42**, 281 (1994)
8 Dwivedi S and Agarwal M P: *J Assoc Physicians India* **42**, 287 (1994)
9 Chopra, B: *J Assoc Physicians India* **42**, 756 (1994)

Tylophora indica

Also known as *Tylophora asthmatica*.

Sanskrit	Anthrapachaka
English	Country Ipecac, Indian Ipecac
Family	Asclepiadaceae
Part Used	Leaves

A perennial branching climber with long fleshy roots occurring in forests of Southern and Eastern India. Could be described as the "Indian Lobelia".

Active Constituents

Alkaloids (0.2 to 0.3%), including tylophorine and tylophorinine.

OCH_3

OCH_3

OCH_3

Tylophorine OCH_3

Pharmacology

- The alkaloids are irritant to the skin and cause nausea and emesis.

- The alkaloids are also toxic to protozoa — hence its use in dysentery, analagous to Ipecac.
- Tylophora extract and its alkaloids have some antitumour activity.[1,2]
- Tylophorine is anti-inflammatory and produces CNS depression in high doses.[3]
- Tylophora has short-lived bronchodilator activity, but this is probably not the basis of the effects in asthma.
- Studies show that the antiasthma effects are more likely to be mediated through depressing cell-mediated immunity:
  - Lymphocyte and eosinophil reduction correlated with prevention of experimentally-induced asthma.[4]
  - Tylophora demonstrated a pronounced inhibition of cell-mediated immunity in mice as evidenced by the increased survival time of skin grafts.[5]
- Tylophorine also stimulates adenylate cyclase in leukcocytes isolated from asthmatic children but not normal children or adults. This represents a stimulation of β-receptor activity.[6]
- Recently it was shown that extracts of Tylophora stimulate the adrenal cortex, increase plasma steroid levels and antagonise steroid-induced suppression of adrenal activity.[7]
- Pure tylophorine is quite toxic with an oral LD50 of 35 mg/kg in rats.[8]

Clinical Studies

- Several trials using one leaf (150 mg/day) for 6 days showed prolonged relief in allergic asthma and rhinitis for up to 12 weeks. (This regime follows traditional use where a sustained effect is obtained from dosing for a short period).[9] This sustained effect may be due to a suppression of the function of helper T cells involved the pathophysiology of asthma.
- In 2 cross-over double blind clinical trials, Tylophora (350 mg/day for 7 days) demonstrated greater symptomatic improvement in patients with bronchial asthma patients than placebo. No significant difference was observed between Tylophora and an antiasthmatic drug, however Tylophora had a more gradual and longer-lasting effect.[10]
- For one trial in asthma results were not significant, but did show a tendency to improvement.[11]
- A study in 1980 on asthma showed that 200 mg/day of Tylophora leaf significantly improved parameters of lung function and depressed eosinophil count.[12]

Adverse Effects

Nausea and vomiting may occur, even at a low dose, especially if the fresh leaves are used.

Actions

Antiasthmatic, anti-inflammatory, immunodepressant, antiallergic.

Medicinal Uses

- Asthma and hayfever as a symptomatic treatment.
- Amoebic dysentery and other protozoal infections.
- As an immune-depressing agent in autoimmune disease.

Dosage

200 to 400 mg/day of the dried herb or 1 to 2 mL/day of the 1:5 tincture. Use short-term intermittent treatment — up to 4 weeks at a time. A convenient dosage regime is 2 mL of the 1:5 tincture for the first 10 days of each calendar month.

REFERENCES

1   Chitnis, M P et al: *Ind J Med Res* **60**, 359 (1972)
2   Donaldson, G R et al: *Biochem Biophys Res Comm* **31**, 104 (1968)
3   Gopalakrishnan, C et al: *Ind J Med Res* **69**, 513 (1979)
4   Haranath, P S R K and Shyamalakumari, S: *Ind J Med Res* **63**, 661 (1975)
5   Atal, C K et al: *J Ethnopharmacol* **18**, 133 (1986).
6   Raina, V and Raina, S: *Biochem Biophys Res Comm* **94**, 1074 (1980)
7   Udupa, A L et al: *Planta Med* **57**, 409 (1991)
8   Dikshith, T S S et al: *Ind J Exp Biol* **28**, 208 (1990)
9   Shivpuri, D N et al: *Annals of Allergy* **30**, 407 (1972)
10 Thiruvengadam K V et al: *J.I.M.A Advertiser* **71**, 170 (1978)
11 Gupta, S et al: *Ind J Med Res* **69**, 981 (1979)
12 Gore, K V et al: *Ind J Med Res* **71**, 144 (1980)

Withania somnifera

Sanskrit	Ashwaghanda
English	Winter Cherry or "Indian Ginseng"
Family	Solanaceae
Part Used	Root

Found in the drier parts of subtropical India and is widely distributed. Also grows in Middle-Eastern countries. Erect shrub up to 1.25 m. Simple leaves up to 10 cm long. Inconspicuous pale green flower in cymes. Fruit is a berry which is orange-red when mature (hence the English name).

Active Constituents[1,2]

- Alkaloids (such as isopelietierine and anaferine).
- Steroidal lactones (withanolides, withaferins).
- Saponins containing an additional acyl group (sitoindoside VII, VIII).
- Withanolides containing a glucose at carbon 27 (sitoindoside IX, X).

Withanolides are also present in leaves and berries. Withania is also rich in iron.[3]

Withanolides

Withaferin A

	R
Sitoindoside IX	H
Sitoindoside X	palmitoyl

Pharmacology — Isolated Constituents

- In high doses alkaloids from Withania exhibited prolonged hypotensive, brady-cardic and respiratory stimulant actions and had a depressant effect on higher cerebral centres.[4] Sedative effects have also been demonstrated.[5]

- Withania alkaloids lower body temperature in mice, have low toxicity, are non-irritant to mucous membranes[6] and are only mild pharmacological agents.

- Withania alkaloids are spasmolytic for intestinal, uterine, bronchial and arterial smooth muscle, with a similar mode of action to papaverine.[5]

- Steroidal compounds in Withania have antibacterial, antitumour and anti-inflammatory activities and some have been shown to protect against carbon tetrachloride induced liver damage.[7] They enhance liver glycogen stores in a similar way to glucocorticoids.[8]

- Withaferin A demonstrated immunosuppressive effects, in contrast to immu-nostimulating activity found for Withania extracts.[9]

- Sitoindosides (VII, VIII, IX, X) protected rats against stress-induced stomach ulcers. An antidepressant effect was observed after the ip administration of sitoindosides VII and VIII to mice subjected to the swimming test.[9,10] Oral administration of sitoindosides IX and X have demonstrated marked improve-ment in learning and memory abilities in mice as well as improvements in both short-term and long-term memory.[9]

Pharmacology — Whole Root

→ Adaptogenic and Tonic Effects

- Young rats were fed Withania or *Asparagus racemosa* at oral doses of 100mg/g for 8 months and observed for body weight, general condition, number of preg-nancies and health of progeny.[8] Weight gain for Withania-treated rats was 227% compared to 159% for Asparagus, and 145% for controls. Animals were alert and in good health. While there was no difference for number and size of preg-nancies, average body-weight of off-spring was 70g for Withania compared to 45g for controls. This study was followed up with a second short-term study over 4 weeks at 250mg/g on adult rats.[8] No weight gain was seen, which indi-cates that Withania's anabolic effect is only exerted in the growth phase. How-ever, other interesting effects in this short-term study were noted. Body temperature was reduced by 1.7 degrees Celsius (reduced metabolic rate?) and liver weight increased in the Withania group. Plasma cortisol was also signifi-cantly lowered and adrenal weight reduced following Withania treatment.[8]

- Several herbs including Withania were evaluated for their protective effects against cyclophosphamide neutropenia in mice.[11] The dosage used was 100 mg/

kg, given for 15 days prior to a single dose of cyclophosphamide and then for 7 days after. Results are tabulated below.

		Day 0	Day 3
Control	Total Count	7800	4390
	Neutrophils	3960	1440
Withania	Total Count	11180	8030
	Neutrophils	7020	5060

Withania significantly increased white blood cell and neutrophil counts both before and after treatment with cyclophosphamide.

Note: Day 3 gave lowest counts. There were no deaths in Withania group compared with 10% mortality in other groups including controls.[11]

- The body weight loss induced by adjuvant arthritis was corrected by 1000mg/Kg Withania given orally over 15 days.[12] Some of inflammation and bony degenerative changes were also decreased.[12]

- At an oral dose of 200 mg/kg in rats, Withania countered many of the biochemical changes of cold stress and immobilisation stress such as rises in blood sugar, lactic acid, urea and creatinine. It did not however counteract the decrease in thymus, liver and kidney weights, but it did somewhat counteract the increase in adrenal weight.[13]

- Seeds of Withania (100 mg/kg, ip) showed a sparing effect on stress-induced adrenal cortisol and ascorbic acid depletion and on adrenal weight increase. They also showed protective effects against aspirin- and stress-induced ulcers. An anabolic effect at oral doses of 100 mg/kg was also demonstrated.[14]

- A recent pharmacological comparison of Withania and *Panax ginseng* demonstrated that Withania had similar potency to Panax in terms of adaptogenic, tonic and anabolic effects.[15]

➡️ *Anti-inflammatory Activity*

- The effect of Withania on experimentally-induced granuloma in rats was compared to cortisone and phenylbutazone. Withania was the most effective in decreasing the glycosaminoglycan content of the granuloma.[16]

- Alpha-2-macroglobulin is a liver-synthesized plasma protein which increases markedly during inflammation. Withania was found to be more effective at decreasing this protein during inflammation when compared to standard anti-inflammatory drugs.[17]

- An anti-inflammatory effect on granuloma tissue formation in rats was observed using an extract of the aerial parts of Withania.[18] The effect was comparable to that achieved by the use of 5 mg/kg hydrocortisone and was believed to be due to the presence of withaferin A.[18]

→ *Antitumour Activity*

- Withania given at 200 mg/kg (whole plant) orally to mice significantly decreased mortality from urethane-induced lung cancers.[19] It increased body weight and countered the decrease in body weight due to the tumours. Withania also decreased incidence, number and size of tumours.[19]

- Withania root extract was administered by ip injection (200–1000 mg/kg/day for 15 days) to mice inoculated with sarcoma cells.[20] Doses of 400 mg/kg and above produced complete regression of tumour after initial growth. The percentage of complete response increased with increasing herb dose although some mortality was observed at the 1000 mg/kg level. Daily doses of 500–750 mg/kg produced a good response.[20]

- A study investigating the effects of Withania, gamma radiation and hyperthermia on sarcoma in mice found Withania (500 mg/kg/day for 10 days, ip administration) produced an 18% rate of complete response.[21] Although the radiation and heat treatments had a greater individual effect on the tumours, Withania increased the effect of these treatments on tumour regression and growth delay when administered concomitantly. The study concluded that Withania had a tumour inhibitory effect and acted as a radiosensitizer.[21]

Clinical Studies

- Withania (2 g/day for 60 days) given in milk significantly increased body weight, total plasma proteins, mean corpuscular haemoglobin and hand grip in a double blind trial on 58 normal children (8–12 years old).[3] The fortified milk was recommended for all age groups especially for young children.[3]

- In a double blind clinical trial, Withania (3 g/day for 1 year) was tested on the process of ageing in 101 healthy male adults (50–59 years old).[22] A significant improvement in haemoglobin, red blood cell count, hair melanin and seated stature was observed. Serum cholesterol decreased and nail calcium was preserved. Eryrocyte sedimentation rate decreased significantly and 71.4% of those treated with the herb reported improvement in sexual performance.[22]

Actions

Tonic, adaptogen, nervine sedative, anti-inflammatory, antitumour (in high doses).

Medicinal Uses

Important tonic because rather than being over-stimulating, Withania has a sedative aspect. Therefore it is very good for people who are "stressed-out". Often combined with Long Pepper to increase its tonic effects.

- Debility, nervous exhaustion especially due to stress.
- Emaciation especially in children, and anaemia.
- Convalescence after acute illness or extreme stress.
- Chronic diseases especially if inflammatory in nature, e.g. connective tissue diseases.
- Impotence due to devitalization.
- May have some preventative role in cancer, especially the whole plant or leaves.
- Good general tonic for disease prevention in athletes, elderly and during pregnancy.

Dosage

3 to 6 g/day or equivalent of the dried root or 6 to 12 mL of 1:2 fluid extract.

REFERENCES

1   Atal, C K et al: *Pharmacognosy and Phytochemisty of Withania somnifera*, CCRIMH, New Delhi (1975)
2   Wagner, H et al: *Phytomedicine* **1**, 63 (1994)
3   Venkatraghavan, S et al: *J Res Ayu Sid* **1**, 370 (1980)
4   Malhotra, C L et al: *Ind J Med Res* **49**, 448 (1961)
5   Malhotra, C L et al: *Ind J Physiol Pharmacol* **9**, 9 (1965)
6   Malhotra, C L et al: *Ind J Physiol Pharmacol* **9**, 127 (1965)
7   Singh, N et al: *Quart J Drug Res* **16**, 8 (1978)
8   Kurandikar et al: *Ind Drugs* **23,** 133 (1986)
9   Ghosal, S et al: *Phytotherapy Res* **3**, 201 (1989) quoted in Wagner, H et al: *Phytomedicine* **1**, 63 (1994)
10 Bhattacharya, S K et al: *Phytotherapy Res* **1**, 32 (1987) quoted in Wagner, H et al: *Phytomedicine* **1**, 63 (1994)
11 Thatte, U M et al: *J Postgrad Med* **33**, 185 (1987)
12 Begum, V H and Sadique, J: *Ind J Exp Biol* **26** 877 (1988)
13 Dadkar, V N et al: *Ind J Clin Biochem* **2** 101 (1987)
14 Singh, N et al: *Int J Crude Drug Res* **20** 29 (1982)
15 Grandhi, A et al: *J Ethnopharmacol* **44**, 131 (1994)
16 Begum, V H and Sadique, J: *Biochem Med Metabol Biol* **38**, 272 (1987)
17 Anbalagan, K and Sadique, J: *Int J Crude Drug Res* **23** 177 (1985)
18 al-Hindawi, M K et al: *J Ethnopharmacol* **37**, 113 (1992)
19 Singh, N et al: *Int J Crude Drug Res* **24** 90 (1986)
20 Devi, P U et al: *Ind J Exp Biol* **30**, 169 (1992)
21 Devi, P U et al: *Ind J Exp Biol* **31**, 607 (1993)
22 Kuppurajan, K et al: *J Res Ayu Sid* **1**, 247 (1980)

Index of Actions

A

abortifacient 92, 99
acrid 25, 46, 80
adaptogenic 16, 35, 40, 69, 71, 72, 99, 138, 140
anabolic 44, 138, 139
analgesic 25, 26, 27, 30, 44, 80, 84, 102
androgenic 44
anthelmintic 97
antiageing 18, 47, 49, 50
antiallergic 31, 32, 54, 75, 78, 81, 85, 92, 95, 129
antianaemic 5
antiandrogenic 98
antianginal 121
antianxiety 37
antiarrhythmic 5, 26, 27, 38, 40, 43, 44, 85
antiasthmatic 92, 136
antiatherogenic 31
antibacterial 15, 56, 59, 65, 67, 78, 94, 97, 138
anticancer 39, 71, 84
anticholesterolaemic 111
anticholinergic 30
anticoagulant 63, 67, 77
anticonvulsant 30, 32, 47, 88, 102
antidepressant 71, 138
antidiabetic 116, 117
antidiarrhoeal 30, 56
antidiuretic 36
antiepileptic 31, 76
antifertility 98
antifibrotic 67, 85
antifilarial 128
antifungal 56, 94
antiglaucoma 106
antihaemorrhagic 44, 54
antihydrotic 87

anti-inflammatory 4, 5, 22, 23, 27, 31, 32, 41, 44, 54, 57, 59, 71, 75, 76, 78, 81, 85, 98, 99, 102, 109, 111, 114, 127, 129, 135, 136, 138, 139, 140
antilithic 114
antimalarial 7
antimicrobial 77, 95, 118
antiobesity 111
antioxidant 49, 50, 64, 70, 71, 81, 98, 127
antiparasitical 11, 56
antiplatelet 4, 5, 67, 76, 98, 105, 106, 111, 128
antiproliferative 5, 77
antipyretic 22, 23, 52, 54, 59, 98, 99
antirheumatic 80
antischistosomal 8
antispasmodic 4, 31, 32, 94, 120, 121, 138
antispermatogenic 98
antisweet activity 115
antitumour 14, 15, 16, 22, 50, 77, 105, 135, 138, 140
antitussive 22, 23, 71, 72
antiulcer 22
antiuraemic 59
antiviral 16, 56, 122, 123, 124
astringent 49, 59

B

beta-blocking 120, 121
biological response modifier 16
bitter 7, 11, 21, 25, 27, 29, 34, 43, 46, 49, 50, 52, 55, 62, 75, 78, 80, 99, 106, 129

bladder tonic 114
blood stimulant 3, 25, 52, 62
bradycardic 138
bronchodilating 91, 92, 105
bronchospasmolytic 106

C

cardioprotective 27, 40, 44, 67, 132, 133
cardiotonic 16, 18, 34, 38, 43, 63, 95, 101, 106
choleretic 97, 99, 127, 129
cognition enhancer 32
cold 7, 21, 29, 52, 55, 62, 75, 80
cytotoxic 10, 65, 77, 123

D

debility 50
depurative 118
diaphoretic 21, 23, 118
diuretic 17, 18, 23, 78, 80, 85, 132, 133

E

expectorant 46, 47, 71, 92

F

fibrinolytic 31, 63, 67, 98
free radical scavenging 127

H

haemostatic 44, 52, 56, 59
hepatoprotective 15, 22, 23, 31, 40, 64, 67, 70, 72, 97, 99, 123, 124, 127, 129, 133

Index of Conditions

General Index